GOD'S PURPOSE IN PAIN:
WHY GOD ALLOWS SUFFERING

By

NORM WIELSCH

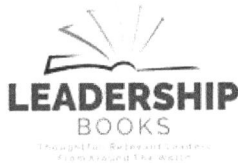

LEADERSHIP
BOOKS
Thoughtful, Relevant Leaders
From Around The World

GODS PURPOSE IN PAIN:

WHY GOD ALLOWS SUFFERING.

By Norm Wielsch

Copyright 2024

Publisher: Leadership Books, Inc.

Las Vegas, Nevada and New York, NY.

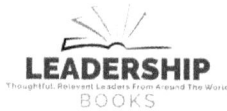

LEADERSHIP

Thoughtful. Relevant Leaders From Around The World

BOOKS

ISBN:

978-1-951648-28-2 (Hardcover)

978-1-951648-58-9 (Paperback)

978-1-951648-59-6 (eBook)

Biblical citations from English Standard Version (ESV)

Printed in the United States of America

DEDICATION

This book was written to those people who have questions about God's sovereignty and love. Your pain has purpose. It is not a coincidence that you are reading this book, it is God's calling upon you. Please accept His calling.

Contents

CHAPTER ONE
INTRODUCTION

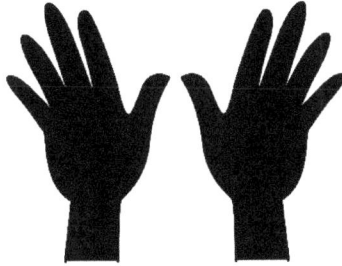

The age-old questions are: Why do bad things happen to good people? Or, why does a loving God allow people to suffer? All this pain and suffering seems so unfair. We ask these questions whenever we enter into an overwhelming life event, heart break, or a traumatic event. Painful life events are no respecters of people. It doesn't matter if you are rich or poor, how much education you have, or what type of job you have – every human will suffer some type of overwhelming life event or traumatic event during their lives. Life's difficult times often come when we least expect them. Some enter into our lives by our own poor decisions and some that we never saw coming. Some trials are more severe than others, but all are painful.

Jesus told us that life would be difficult. What do you do when life becomes overwhelming? You lose your job? Your spouse leaves you. Corona Virus hits your community, have legal and/or financial problems, or diagnoses of an illness.

The question of why God allows suffering is a difficult question to answer. The answers are found in the bible. There are several different reasons–all are difficult to reconcile. But first let's build a foundation. Merriam-Webster defines *suffering* as meaning the state of being in great trouble; implies great physical or mental strain and stress, sickness, poverty, or loss. Suffering can be painful.

Let's begin with some truths of the bible, the first question: Why do bad things happen to good people? This is difficult to explain and even more difficult to understand. But I'm going to try. This is my opinion based on my study of the bible. Why do bad things happen to "good" people? What does the bible say about people? And what is the definition of "good?" God tells us in Genesis 6:5,

> "The LORD saw that the wickedness of man was great in the earth, and that every intention of the thoughts of his [and her] heart was only evil continually."

And the Apostle Paul adds his insight on human nature in his letter to the Romans 3:10-12,

> "...none [no one] is righteous, no, not one; no one understands; no one seeks for God. All have turned aside... no one does good, not even one."

Doctor Luke describes a conversation between a rich man and Jesus. The man called Jesus "good teacher." Jesus replied, "Why do you call me good? No one is good except God alone." The bible teaches that no human being is good (Mark 10:17-22).

Merriam-Webster defines *"good"* as: of favorable character, deserving of respect and honor. The dictionary was written by man. How does society define *"good?"* Is it the same?

What about the term *"bad?"* Merriam-Webster defines *bad* as: unfavorable, unpleasant, or harmful. How does society define "bad?" The same? How does God define these terms? The question then comes up: Can a bad event in our lives be for our good? Can pain make us see our lives from a different perspective and bring understanding, and even produce joy? These questions are deep and debatable. These are questions for the temporal world. Christians are only visitors on this earth. We are citizens of heaven (Philippians 3:20). Our temporal life and experiences here on earth prepare us for our eternal life in heaven.

As Jesus said, "Only God is good." This is an absolute fact. Relatively speaking, some people are better than others. Most people have the tendency to believe they are "more-good" than other people. But God says no human being is good. This is a result of Adam's sin in the Garden of Eden. The Bible teaches that all humans are equally evil. No one is better than anyone else. All sin is equally bad. I hope this makes sense.

Can "bad" things happen to good people? The word "bad" is relative. What is considered bad? A loss of a job? An illness? The death of a loved one? How about winning the lottery? Can sudden wealth be bad? Or, would it be considered bad if you don't have the assurance of eternal life in heaven? How bad can a painful overwhelming life event be when compared to your salvation and living eternally in heaven with God? Should we blame God for ensuring your salvation? Paul says it best in First Corinthians 2:9,

> "What no eye has seen, nor ear heard, nor the heart of man imagined, what God has prepared [in heaven] for those who love Him."

Pain and suffering are common to all inhabitants of earth. Should we pray for God to remove the pain? Does God have a purpose for the pain? If so, should we pray the pain away? Is that going against God's will? Pain is temporal. Our time on this earth is short. Jesus tells us that there is nothing on earth we should fear because He has already overcome the trappings of the world. Our focus should not be on our pain, but on the One who holds the key to the entrance of heaven.

If we accept that it is permissible for God to allow bad things to happen to non-believers who have no salvation – so that they can be saved, the next question becomes: Why do bad things happen to faithful Christians? Have you been a faithful Christian? Have you made Jesus your Lord and Savior? If so, that's good because according to the bible,

> "And we know that for those who love God all things work together for good, for those who are called according to His [God's] purpose." -- Romans 8:28

The answer is: no bad things happen to Christians. All things work together for the good. Even events that bring us pain prepare us for God's Kingdom. Romans 8:29 adds that, God chooses us to be Christians. And those whom He chose, He predestined to be molded into the likeness of Jesus. If you are reading this, God chose you to be a Christian. His will for you is to make you more in the image of His son – even if that involves painful events. God cares more about your soul than your physical body, He does all He can to prepare us for the Kingdom of Heaven.

When we evaluate our painful situation from a human perspective, we may say, "God why me? It's not fair." The term "*fair*" is also relative. What is fair? Merriam-Webster defines "*fair*" as: impartial; free from self-interest, prejudice, or favoritism. Is your sense of fair the same as mine? When we ask, "God, why me?" We tend to blame and become angry at God. We misunderstand God's love; then we ask, "Is this what God thinks of me?" This can be a slippery slope and will lead to low self-worth. God loved you while you were a sinner, He sent His Son to take your place on the cross so that you could be forgiven. His love is unconditional.

King Nebuchadnezzar conquered Israel and took thousands of Jews captive and made them slaves. He was an evil king; he did not acknowledge the God of the Jews. Daniel 4:28-37, tells us that Nebuchadnezzar was filled with pride. He was rich and powerful. One day he was reveling in his great power and majesty. Because of his pride, God intended to humble him and bring him to salvation. God took Nebuchadnezzar's kingdom away. God made it so that the king was like an animal, eating grass like an ox. The Bible says that his hair grew out like eagle's feathers and his fingernails were like bird's claws. After a period of time (some believe years had passed), Nebuchadnezzar acknowledged God's sovereignty. At that time, his sanity returned to him. After repenting, his kingdom was restored, and his majesty and splendor returned to him. Nebuchadnezzar said, "Now I, Nebuchadnezzar, praise and extol and honor the King of Heaven, for all His works are right and His ways are just, and those who walk in pride He is able to humble" Daniel 4:37.

Everything was taken from King Nebuchadnezzar; he was forced to live in the wilderness for years. He went from the palace to the pit. But he still maintained that God was fair and just. His pain brought him a different perspective and produced joy.

God is fair and just. It is our selfish nature that forces us to see our situation from a worldly perspective. The *"world"* is a societal system that goes against God and is led by Satan. Based on this perspective, or worldview, our sense of fairness is skewed. It is not fairness that is our true concern, but it is our judgment on God's decision how His blessings are distributed. We tend to compare ourselves from a self-centered perspective and think, "I'm better than him/her, but they have a better house or car than I do, it's not fair;" Or, "I'm a good person, why do I have cancer and that drug addict is healthy?" "It's not fair!" We are human and flawed – we always compare ourselves to others. Its human nature. When we cannot make sense of these questions – we blame God.

This way of thinking is as old as humanity. Psalm 73 laments on this subject, the author Asaph, wrote that he lost confidence in God because he was envious of the prosperity of evil people. He saw that people who he considered to be evil lived healthy and wealthy lives, never appearing to have difficult times like the rest. Asaph goes on to say, nevertheless, "I make God my LORD."

This all seems unfair; however, perspective is important here. In Luke 6:19-31, we read about the story of the rich man and Lazarus. Many theologians believe this is a true story because Jesus identifies the poor man by name. Speaking to the religious elite, Jesus told of an unnamed rich man who wore beautiful expensive clothing and ate delicious food, and a poor man named Lazarus who was poor and was covered in sores. Lazarus ate only what fell off the rich man's table. In this story, both men died. Lazarus went to heaven, described as being at Abraham's side (Abraham represents God). The rich man went to hell. As the rich man was being tormented in hell, he was crying out for mercy, asking for just a small amount of water to cool his tongue. Abraham responded to the rich man and said, "Child, remember that you in your lifetime received good things, and Lazarus in like manner bad things; but now he is comforted here, and you are in anguish."

Those who outwardly appear to have everything going for them – may not. The rich man lived a lavish life, the best of everything. He had everything he wanted but never thought of eternity. Lazarus suffered during his life and is now feasting with Jesus and enjoying all the Kingdom of God has to offer. With this perspective, did Lazarus get the short end of the stick? He lived a painful life of need and ridicule – begging for food. But now he is living the good life in heaven. Where would you rather spend eternity?

To make peace in regards to suffering we must acknowledge and understand God's sovereignty. He is on the throne and in control and is a loving and merciful God. He is our creator, our heavenly Father who loves us with the unconditional love that only He can give. We are all God's children, both believers and non-believers. He loves us so much that He allows us to experience pain so that we will know joy. He allows us to be broken so we know what it feels like to be healed. When you understand and accept that God is in charge, the pressure is off. You will stop trying to control and manipulate your situation. Give your pain to God – trust Him. Jeremiah 29:11 says,

> "For I [God] know the plans I have for you, declares the LORD, plans for welfare and not for evil, to give you a future and a hope."

It is imperative that we believe and trust God's promises, especially the promise that all things will work for the good for those who love God.

It is all perspective; life on earth is temporary. We need to set our sights on the Kingdom of Heaven. I know that this mind-set is not easy to achieve. I've had my share of pain and suffering, but each time that I trusted in God, He walked with me hand-in-hand. Sometimes He had to carry me, but I made it through and came out better for it.

When we understand that God is our creator, and we His creation; we see that God's love for His creation is indescribable. We can see that God strategically and thoughtfully allows, orchestrates and ordains trials in our lives for our own good and the good of His kingdom. This is a difficult concept to comprehend, but once understood, it will bring peace, contentment, and joy into your life.

Most people falsely believe that once you become a Christian, you never have to endure another painful emotional or physical trial. This is a distorted and simplistic view of God. The truth is, Christians will be subjected to difficult times in life. Jesus promised that He will help us through our painful times. Remember, God chose you and has a plan and purpose for your life. Any painful experience that comes into your life, God allowed, and its purpose is to prepare you for heaven.

We should never deny the place of pain and suffering in building godliness in the Christian life. Though there is much needless pain we bear through lack of knowledge and consequences of our sin, there is also necessary suffering. If suffering was how the Father taught Jesus, is it not a suitable tool to teach us?

We often do not understand the purpose for the pain. But parents understand, we must allow our children to endure painful events for their own good. Like an infant who must be immunized, the immunization benefits the infant preventing disease. The injection is painful, the child does not understand the reason for the pain, but it is for their own good. They don't like it, but they need it to become a healthy adult. God allows us to experience pain for our own good so that we will be spiritually healthy.

All humans have one thing in common, we will all go through trials and traumatic painful events. When a non-believer goes through a trial, they only see the painful situation. No purpose to the pain. Christians who go through trials look at the trial through a Christian worldview – the pain has a purpose. Romans 5:3-5 says,

> "...we rejoice in our sufferings, knowing that suffering produces endurance, and endurance produces character, and character produces hope, and hope does not put us to shame, because God's love has been poured out into our hearts through the Holy Spirit who has been given to us."

God wants you to persevere through trials, when you do, you fulfill God's plan for your life, to mold you into the likeness of Jesus. When everything is going good in our lives, we become self-sufficient, we fail to rely on God for everything in life. We become our own god. We do not grow or mature as a Christian. It is only through adversity and pain that change and growth is produced.

A great example of how pain produces something good is the example of the pearl. A pearl is beautiful, valuable, and desired; but it doesn't come easy. Imagine you are an oyster sitting on the bottom of the ocean. You're minding your own business enjoying the relaxing motion of the water. When you least expect it, a grain of sand gets into your shell. This grain of sand represents a trial in your life. If you look at a grain of sand under a microscope you would see that it has jagged edges. The grain of sand scrapes against the inside of your shell and irritates you to your soul. The sharp edges cause discomfort and pain. Oysters don't have hands so they cannot remove the sand. An oyster will secrete a substance that coats the grain of sand in an attempt to stop the pain. But the pain does not stop. The oyster secretes more and more of this substance in a continual effort to coat the grain to stop the pain. However, there is still no relief to the pain. We do the same thing; we try everything we can to remove the pain. But this process continues until the substance eventually forms a pearl. The pain that the oyster endured becomes a beautiful pearl. No matter what we do or who we manipulate, we cannot remove our pain until God's work is complete in us. There was a purpose to the pain.

I don't know what you have been through or going through right now. Maybe you had a difficult childhood, had a dream or a plan for your life that was snatched away from you, or you have been diagnosed with a debilitating disease, or something much worse. Some of these situations were out of your control, some may be consequences of poor decisions or choices, we can all relate to these circumstances. There are hundreds of different types of trials of varying intensities. Know that God is with you in your pain. God is on the throne and allowed your pain. Whether Satan orchestrated the evil or it was a result of your own doing, God has a plan to work your pain for your good. When you accept that God is sovereign and in control and you praise Him through your painful trial, you will come out understanding God's work in your life – you will see God's fingerprints all over your pain. God is working something good in you, just like the oyster and pearl, pain can bring beauty.

Each trial is an opportunity for growth. It is all about perspective. How we feel and talk about our trial sets the tone. When we complain and blame others, we magnify our pain and this often extends the duration of the pain. Our attitude transforms from being angry and bitter to being grateful that God loves us so much that He wants to make us better.

God does not owe anyone an explanation; we are not entitled to an explanation. There is nothing in scripture that says He will give us a reason for His decisions. The life events that we go through are not by accident; they are by providence. They are essential to our growth and training.

Is eliminating pain a loving thing to do? If we love someone, do we allow them to do anything they want? Treat people poorly? No boundaries or rules? No moral standards? Would this be your parenting philosophy?

Why would God create a world that has suffering? Is it possible that character issues can only be refined through adversity? Is it only through adversity that we learn to empathize with others by experiencing pain ourselves? Some of our greatest lessons are learned through trials. So, can we say that pain is not an indicator of whether something is beneficial?

Your trial is not an accident or just bad luck, there is no such thing as coincidences. God is in control. He knows what you are going through, He allowed it! He would never have allowed it if He wasn't going to work it for your own good. Let's read about what the bible says about suffering.

CHAPTER TWO
WHO IS GOD?

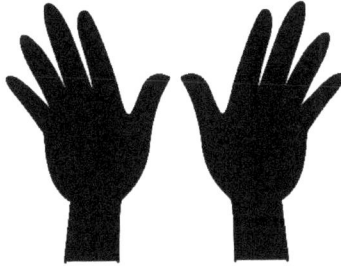

"Thus says the LORD who made you, who formed you from the womb and will help you… 'I will pour my Spirit upon your offspring, and My blessing on your descendants…' Thus says the LORD, the King of Israel and His Redeemer, the LORD of Hosts: 'I am the first and I am the last; besides Me there is no god.'" --Isaiah 44:2 -2, 6

All people on earth, at some level, have an inner sense that there is a God – creator of the universe exists. The Apostle Paul says,

"For the wrath of God is revealed from heaven against all ungodliness and unrighteousness of men, who by their unrighteousness suppress the truth. For what can be known about God is plain to them, because God has shown it to them. For His invisible attributes, namely, His eternal power and divine nature, have been clearly perceived, ever since the creation of the world, in the things that have been made. So, they are without excuse. For although they knew God, they did not honor Him as God or give thanks to Him, but they became futile in their thinking, and their foolish hearts were darkened. Claiming to be wise, they became fools, and exchanged the glory of the immortal God for images resembling mortal man and birds and animals and creeping things. Therefore, God gave them up in the lusts of their hearts to impurity, to the dishonoring of their bodies among themselves, because they exchanged the truth about God for a lie and worshiped and served the creature rather than the Creator, who is blessed forever! Amen. For this reason God gave them up to dishonorable passions." -- Romans 1:19-23

All people should know there is a God because they see the beauty of creation. They know in their hearts that creation is not just a gene mutation. But still, some say, "There is no God." Since the fall, everyone born after Adam is born separated from God. Humans were originally created to be in fellowship with God, but now we don't know Him. Since Adam's sin, we were born with a hole in our hearts, we search for something to fill that hole. We spend our entire lives searching for something -- anything to fill that void. We try to fill it with material things: wealth, power, status, alcohol and/or drugs, relationships, or other addictive behavior. We thought that these behaviors would satisfy us. They may have made us feel good in the short term, but we soon find they did not give us the peace we were looking for. Nothing will fill that void because it is God-shaped.

It is only through making Jesus Christ your Lord and Savior that the hole in your heart will be filled, and you will be made whole.

Belief in an almighty loving creator is not based on blind hope with no evidence. Two proofs of evidence of a heavenly creator are:

1) Everything in the universe has a cause; everything works together and has a purpose. This is not by accident, Colossians 1:15-17 says,

> "He [Jesus] is the image of the invisible God, the firstborn of all creation. For by Him all things were created, in heaven and on earth, visible and invisible, whether thrones or dominions or rulers or authorities— all things were created through Him and for Him. And He is before all things, and in Him all things hold together."

Jesus holds all created things together. Without Him there is chaos.

2) Right and wrong. We are in a moral dilemma, the world is sinful, but God wrote the sense of right and wrong on our hearts.

> "For this is the covenant that I [God] will make with the house of Israel after those days, declares the LORD: I will put my law within them, and I will write it on their hearts. And I will be their God, and they shall be my people." --Jeremiah 31:33

In order for a society to exist, there must be a justice system. Can an immoral society controlled by Satan judge right from wrong? In this type of a system, can there be a moral standard? Who will judge good and evil? I believe that without God, there is no fair judgment for right and wrong. There must be a just God that has the authority to forgive humanity for its sins.

If these two reasons are true, why don't all people believe? Because since the fall, Satan has control of the earth, 2 Corinthians 4:4 tells us that Satan has control of the earth and that he has blindfolded the eyes of non-believers from understanding the gospel of Jesus Christ. There is an unseen spiritual war going on all around us – good vs evil. God is the only one who can remove this blindfold so that the saving grace of the gospel can be understood.

Humans are finite, God is infinite. Psalm 147:5 says, "Great is our LORD, and abundant in power, His understanding is beyond measure." To know God, we must understand who God is. His attributes include:

1) God is omnipresent – God is not limited to space and time; He is in every place in the heavens and on earth at the same time; there is no place that He is not.

2) God is omniscience – God knows everything, past, present, and future; there is nothing He does not know.

3) God is omnipotent – God is sovereign - all powerful, there is nothing He cannot do.

4) God is loving – We are His creation – He loves us unconditionally. His righteousness is tempered with love, patience, mercy, and grace. This attribute sets Him apart from other deities and is the reason we have hope.

5) God is sovereign – God created mankind and has ultimate right to rule as He chooses. He has the right to make the rules, expect His creation to follow them, and to hold His creation accountable for their behavior.

When we understand that God created all things and is all-powerful, it is reasonable to conclude that God directs and holds together all things. The theological term for this is *providence.* Merriam-Webster defines *"providence"* as: divine guidance or the power sustaining and guiding human destiny. Providence says that God is directly involved with His creation where He keeps it in existence, maintains its properties, and directs them to act as they do – all this to fulfill His plan and purpose.

God is interested in and active in all aspects of your life. God causes events in your lives to occur. For example: God placed this book in your hands, it was not an accident that you are reading it right now. There are no coincidences in this life – God is actively involved. He knows you intimately, and He knows how many hairs are on your head, He knows what you need before you think you need it. God gave humans the freedom to choose to follow Him or not. You are free to choose your own way in life. However, God's plan and purpose in your life supersede your plans. Proverbs explains this,

- "Commit your work to the LORD, and your plans will be established." --Proverbs 16:3

- "The LORD has made everything for its purpose, even the wicked for the day of trouble." --v. 16:4

- "When a man's ways please the LORD, he makes even his enemies to be at peace with him." --v. 16:7

- "The heart of man plans his way, but the LORD establishes his steps." --v.16:9

- "There is a way that seems right to a man, but its end is the way to death." --v.16:25

We are free to make our own decisions – the problem is that without God; and left to our own devices, we will fail. Again, because of the fall, our heart seeks to go against God. God says that our hearts are desperately corrupt (Jeremiah 17:9) and that nothing good lives in us (Romans 7:18). There are good people (depending on your definition of good), but we all fall short of God's moral standards.

God chooses those who He wants to spend eternity with Him in heaven. He made the choice before He created the heavens and earth (Ephesians 1:4). The term for this is election which is defined as an act of God where He chooses some people to be saved. Not by anything good or bad that we had done, but only through God's grace and mercy. First Thessalonians 1:4-5 says,

> "For we know, brothers loved by God, that He has chosen you, because our gospel came to you not only in

word, but also in power and in the Holy Spirit and with full conviction."

And 2 Thessalonians 2:13-14 adds,

> "But we ought always to give thanks to God for you, brothers beloved by the LORD, because God chose you as the firstfruits to be saved, through sanctification by the Spirit and belief in the truth. To this He called you through our gospel, so that you may obtain the glory of our LORD Jesus Christ."

If you are reading this book, congratulations – you've been chosen by God to be saved! Understanding this concept is extremely important because your peace and joy come from who God is and who you are in-Christ. The creator of the universe chose you to live with Him for eternity. You may now praise Him for what He has done in your life, go ahead, I'll wait. Don't let pride overcome you, He chose you not because you did or will do something good, He chose you because of His grace and mercy.

Some people sadly believe, "God could never choose me, I've made too many mistakes and too many bad choices in my life." This way of thinking could not be further from the truth, First Corinthians 1:26-29 says,

> "For consider your calling, brothers: not many of you were wise according to worldly standards, not many were powerful, not many were of noble birth. But God chose what is foolish in the world to shame the wise; God chose

what is weak in the world to shame the strong; God chose what is low and despised in the world, even things that are not, to bring to nothing things that are, so that no human being might boast in the presence of God."

God chooses those who have been-there-and-done-that. That includes making bad decisions, making mistakes, and those who have been marginalized and neglected. He has a plan and purpose for every person. He chose you for your potential.

In the Old Testament, there was a Jewish man named Gideon (Judges chapters 6 – 8). The Midianites and Israelites were enemies. The Midianites were attacking Israel. Gideon was hiding in a winepress to avoid detection of the Midianites. An angel of the LORD appeared to him and said, "The LORD is with you, O mighty man of valor." Gideon was not acting like a mighty man, or a man of valor. The angel sent from God knew of Gideon's potential. God chose Gideon to defeat the Midianite army. Gideon defeated the enemy even though they were outnumbered. Gideon's potential was to be a mighty man of valor, you are too!

You have a unique sphere of influence that others do not have. You can reach people that I could never influence. God does not make mistakes – He chose you to serve Him. God is a spirit. He needs humans to fulfill His will on earth. We are His workers. Don't worry about your past, you are more than a conqueror through Jesus who gives you the power to be victorious. God chose you, be honored.

God has a plan and purpose for our lives. God gives each person the gifts and abilities to fulfill that plan to benefit God's kingdom. These abilities are often obtained by going through painful trials. When we come out of the trial better than before, we have the ability to help others going through similar trials. God will place us in situations where we can be a help to others. It is your choice to help or to ignore someone suffering. If you ignore your calling, God will get someone else to do it. You can accept God's calling the easy way or the hard way. Believe me, the hard way is not fun.

A great example in the bible of our freedom of choice is in the story of Jonah. Second Kings 14:25 talks about the Prophet Jonah. Jesus also mentioned Jonah in Matthew chapter twelve. If Jesus talked about Jonah and the great fish and what happened, that is good enough for me.

The story is set in 760 B.C.., during this time, the city of Nineveh was the capitol of Assyria. The people in the city were evil in God's eyes, they hated the Israelites and were idolaters. God called on the Jewish prophet Jonah to go to Nineveh and preach repentance to them. If they would not repent, God said He would destroy the city. Jonah hated the Assyrians because of their cruelty to the Jewish people. Jonah wanted God to destroy the city and all the people in it. He did not want the people to repent and be saved. Nineveh was about 500 miles from Jerusalem where he lived. Jonah refused God's calling, he chose to go against God's calling and went to a coastal town and got on a ship heading the opposite direction. He headed to Tarshish, which was 2,500 miles in the opposite direction as

Nineveh. I don't know what he was thinking, no one can escape God's presence. God had another plan.

When the ship got out to sea, God brought up a great wind, so strong that the ship was breaking apart. The ship's brave crew became frightened. They each cried out to their own god for help, but none of their gods came to their aid. They began to throw cargo overboard to lighten the load. Where was Jonah? In the hull of the ship sleeping. The captain woke Jonah and ordered him to pray to his God for help. I often wonder how many gods were prayed to that day. The crew began to cast lots to determine who was responsible for the storm. During that time, casting lots was a way to determine who God chose regarding whatever they were deciding. Small stones were placed in a bag or jar, one stone was marked. Each individual would pull out a stone, the person who picked the marked stone was the person God chose. Jonah chose the marked stone, this indicated that Jonah was responsible for the storm.

The men questioned Jonah, who admitted that he was running away from God. The storm grew stronger, the crew asked Jonah how they could calm the storm. Jonah said, "Pick me up and hurl me into the sea; then the sea will quiet down for you…" They did not want to throw Jonah overboard, but as the storm grew stronger, they decided it was the only way to save everyone. They threw Jonah into the raging sea. The storm then calmed down. The ship's crew now believed in Jonah's God – the God of Israel. The crew made sacrifices to God and vowed to follow Him.

Scripture says, "...the LORD appointed a great fish to swallow up Jonah." The text tells us that he was in the belly of the fish for three days and three-nights. The writer does not go into specifics about what type of fish it was. After three days, Jonah prayed to God, repented, and submitted to God's will. The fish then spit him out onto land. God called out to Jonah again, "Arise and go to Nineveh, that great city, and call out against it the message that I tell you." Jonah submitted and went to Nineveh. The fish had placed him about 60 miles or a three-day journey from Nineveh.

When Jonah reached Nineveh, he preached God's word to repent their sins or be destroyed. The people believed him and repented, even the king repented. When God saw that the people repented, He relented on His punishment. More than 120,000 people were saved that day.

Jonah should have been happy, but he had a deep-rooted hatred for the people of this city. Jonah was angry at God for not killing all the people in the city. Jonah said,

> "...O LORD, is not this what I said when I was yet in my country? That is why I made haste to flee to Tarshish; for I knew that you are a gracious God and merciful, slow to anger and abounding in steadfast love, and relenting from disaster. Therefore now, O LORD, please take my life from me, for it is better for me to die than to live." -- Jonah 4:2-3

Jonah preferred to die than to see these people be reconciled to God. Jonah walked outside the city and built himself a shelter.

He intended to wait to see if God would destroy the city. He had forgotten how God showed mercy on him when he rebelled, why could he not do the same for the people of Nineveh? God created a plant to grow next to the shelter to provide some shade from the heat of the sun. Jonah was happy to have some shade, but the next day God allowed a worm to eat and kill the plant. The temperature increased and God brought up a great wind causing Jonah to overheat and become faint. Jonah became angry at the plant and God. He asked God to let him die. God asked him if it felt good to be angry at a plant. Jonah replied that it did and said he was angry enough to die.

God responded saying that Jonah pitied the plant. He did not plant its seed nor watered it, God created it. The story ends with God asking why Jonah could not pity the people of the city of Nineveh because they were spiritually lost.

God used the plant to teach Jonah a lesson – God is sovereign. Because of his selfish motivations, he was angry at the plant. But he would not give the death of hundreds of thousands of people a second thought. The people of Nineveh were God's children, He loves all His children. God does what He wills, but He is patient; waiting for His children to repent. We don't know what happened to Jonah after the story ends, if he learned a lesson about who God is, or not. This story gives us an excellent example of what happens when you run from God's calling. Jonah chose the hard way over the easy way. He could have just as easily went to Nineveh and preached God's word and fulfilled God's will. If you hear God's calling, what will you do?

Jeremiah was a prophet of God. God wanted to teach Jeremiah about His sovereignty in regards to the Nation of Israel. Jeremiah 18:1-4 says,

> "The word that came to Jeremiah from the LORD: Arise, and go down to the potter's house, and there I will let you hear my words. So, I [Jeremiah] went down to the potter's house, and there he [potter] was working at his wheel. And the vessel he was making of clay was spoiled in the potter's hand, and he reworked it into another vessel, as it seemed good to the potter to do."

In order to obtain true peace in life, we must acknowledge that God is the creator of all things. God compared himself to a clay potter – a divine potter. We are His creation – His clay. As does the potter, God has the ultimate right as our creator to mold us into His vision. He molds us each uniquely different. Different shapes, sizes, colors, abilities, gifts, personalities, and characters. Every person on earth is a child of God – a wonderful work of art. How can anyone ask, "Why have you made me like this?" You are exactly as God intended. If God wanted you to have a different nose, chin, skin color, or hair color, He would have given them to you.

The prophet Isaiah was taught God's sovereignty:

> "Thus says the LORD, your Redeemer, who formed you from the womb: 'I am the LORD, who made all things, who alone stretched out the heavens, who spread out the earth by Myself, who frustrates the signs of liars and

makes fools of diviners, who turns wise men back and makes their knowledge foolish…'" --Isaiah 44:24-25

"I am the LORD, and there is no other, besides Me there is no God; I equip you, though you do not know Me, that people may know, from the rising of the sun and from the west, that there is none besides Me; I am the LORD, and there is no other. I form light and create darkness; I make well-being and create calamity; I am the LORD, who does all these things." --v. 45:5-7

"For thus says the LORD, who created the heavens (He is God!), who formed the earth and made it (He established it; He did not create it empty, He formed it to be inhabited!): 'I am the LORD, and there is no other.'" --v. 45:18

God created all things. Paul tells us that all things were created through Jesus Christ and for him all things are held together (Colossians 1:15-16). Everything God creates has a purpose. He governs and directs all things so that His purpose will be accomplished.

God holds all things together and maintains them as He seems fit. God is involved in every aspect of life in this world. He has a plan and purpose for every person; whether you believe in Him or not. It is your own choice to follow him – or not. If you make the choice to go your own way, you will never experience the peace and joy that a relationship with God will bring.

If God is intimately involved in our lives and loves us, so why is there evil? Evil is a result of the fall. God did not create evil; evil is a result of Satan's rule in this world. But God does use evil to fulfill His purposes. He knows the hearts of all people who will eventually come to Him, and who will not. God knows the bigger picture; He can use an inherently evil person to bring about good. An example is the pharaoh who enslaved the Israelites.

Due to their idolatry, the Israelites were enslaved in Egypt for 400 years. In the story of the Exodus, God chose Moses to deliver His people out of the oppression of Egypt. Moses spoke to pharaoh several times asking to release God's people. The pharaoh refused each request. God, in order to convince the pharaoh of His power, brought ten plagues; one-at-a-time upon entire Egypt. After each plague Moses asked the pharaoh to release the people. After several plagues, pharaoh was eager to free the Israelites. The bible says that, "God hardened the heart of pharaoh" (14:8). The pharaoh changed his mind and refused to release the Israelites. The question comes up: We have freedom of choice, but doesn't God control us as He did the pharaoh? God's hardening of the pharaoh's heart was a response to pharaoh's own evil heart. If the pharaoh knew the God of Israel, he would have released the slaves. Why would God influence a person to make such a decision? Why not just influence pharaoh to agree to let the people go and be done with it? Exodus 9:16 says,

> "But for this purpose, I [God] have raised you [pharaoh] up, to show you my power, so that my name may be proclaimed in all the earth."

Because of God's miracles in Egypt including the defeat of pharaoh's great army reinforced belief in the God of Israel; and showed the rest of the world that the God of Israel is the one true living God. It is true that many people had to suffer and die during the ten plagues. However, the number of believers saved as a result of this event cannot be underestimated. The testimony of both the Egyptians and the Israelites brought many more to God.

There is nothing on earth that God is not in control of. That means either God allows pain and suffering or He ordains it. It was God's divine plan of salvation that required His Son to be crucified on the cross. That meant that Jesus was required to suffer emotional and physical pain and die a slow death on the cross. You may ask, "Why would a loving God allow His own Son to be beaten and murdered? It is because of God's uncomprehendable love for us that He sacrificed His only Son. It is only through Jesus' death and resurrection that the world could be forgiven and saved from the torment of hell.

God uses all things and people to fulfill His purpose for you, your family, and the Kingdom of God. The secret to having peace in times of trouble is to understand the principle that God is sovereign and in control. When you go through an overwhelming life event, rest assured that God is on the throne and in control. Romans 8:28 says,

"And we know that for those who love God all things work together for good, for those who are called according to His purpose."

When we believe that everything happens for our good for those who love God – we can weather any storm because we know God is in control. He will never allow any more pain in your life than you can handle. This does not mean the storm will be easy, but it does give you a different perspective on your pain and suffering. A new perspective – a godly perspective. One that changes your prayer from "God, why me? Why are you doing this to me?" To "God, thank you, teach me what you want me to know, I love you."

God is in control and uses painful events to mold you into the likeness of Jesus Christ. Your suffering has a purpose, it is only through painful events that we achieve understanding. No need to worry about anything – God is on the throne.

CHAPTER THREE
THE FALL OF MAN

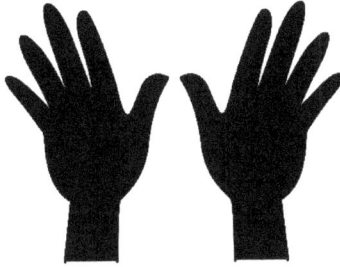

"Therefore, just as sin came into the world through one man, and death through sin, and so death spread to all men because all sinned…" --Romans 5:12

To better understand the question of suffering, we need to know God's intent and design in regard to creation. Genesis chapter 1-3 gives us a historic look at creation of the heavens, earth, and everything living in it. God had a specific intent to create human beings. After He created a home for man to live in, God said, "Let us make man in our image, after our likeness." God breathed life into man; and man became a living creature. God placed His creation (Adam) in the Garden of Eden. The garden grew every plant and tree that looked nice and gave Adam good food. The Tree of Life provided him eternal life, and another tree was called the Tree of Knowledge of Good and Evil.

God put Adam to work in the garden. God commanded Adam not to eat the fruit from the Tree of Knowledge. This came with a warning, God told Adam if he ate from the tree he would die. Adam was allowed to eat from any of the other trees and plants, except the one. This was God's only rule placed on Adam.

God saw that Adam was alone on the earth. God said it was not good for man to be alone. God created a woman from Adam's rib. The union of marriage was now instituted. Adam and Eve lived together in the garden. The Bible says that they were naked but not ashamed of it. God blessed them both and commanded them to procreate and fill the earth with their descendants. God's relationship with the first humans was good, God gave control of the entire earth to Adam and his wife. This was a beautiful time, there was no death because of the Tree of Life. All animals and Adam and Eve were created vegetarians. Flesh was not eaten. God looked at His creation and said it was very good.

Genesis 1:26 says, "Then God said, 'Let us make man in our image, after our likeness." The dictionary defines "image" as an exact likeness, a person strikingly like another person, or a vivid or graphic representation of another. Most theologians believe it refers to the image of the triune God – God the Father, God the Son, and God the Holy Spirit. Humans also have three distinct parts -- flesh, a soul, and a spirit. The flesh is our physical body; the flesh relates to the world through our senses. The soul is the center of our mind, will, emotions, and personality. The spirit was created to be in union with God the Father. In God's image includes being holy, intelligent, with free will, and to have eternal life. These character traits gave them a close personal relationship with God.

Satan was once a high-ranking and beautiful angel (Isaiah 14:12-14 & Ezekiel 28:11-19), I imagine that since God banished Satan to earth, he lost his good looks and is now ugly. Satan committed the very first sin in the universe. His name was originally Lucifer. Lucifer wanted to place himself above God and be God. This was the sin of pride. The consequence for his sin was that God banished him from heaven, forcing him to live on earth.

In Genesis chapter three, we are told about the first sin on earth. One day Eve was enjoying a beautiful day in the garden. She was minding her own business when a serpent approached her. In the bible, serpents or snakes represent Satan. Why a serpent? I don't know, but the scriptures say that the serpent was "more-crafty" that all other animals. Crafty can be defined a swindler or adept in the use of subtlety and cunning. Satan is a cunning creation. If Satan approached Eve in his real form, Eve would have run away. This is why he came to her as something familiar within the garden – a snake.

This is how Satan operates, he attacks us in the form of someone or something we recognize and are comfortable with so that our suspicion is not alerted. Satan is a master at manipulation, trying to get us to doubt our beliefs and understanding; he asked Eve, "Did God actually say, 'You shall not eat of any tree in the garden?'" his statement takes the form of a question. It is genius because it distorts God's word. He suggests that God is withholding something good from the couple. He suggests the thought to her that God was not good, He is unfair, and has too many rules. Eve said that they were allowed to eat from all other plants and trees, except the one; eating from the fruit of the prohibited tree would cause death. Satan said, "You will not surely die. For God knows that when you eat of it your eyes will be opened, and you will be like God, knowing good and evil." Satan is playing on her pride and ego suggesting that God is lying and does not have her best interest in mind. The bible says that when Eve saw that the forbidden fruit was good to eat, beautiful to look at, and was going to make them smart as God - she ate. She gave some to Adam who also ate of the forbidden fruit. First John 2:16 says, "For all that is in the world—the desires of the flesh and the desires of the eyes and pride of life— is not from the Father but is from the world."

This is a perfect model of how Satan operates. We accept Satan's lies that God is withholding good thing from us, so we go out and try to get them ourselves - often by any means necessary. We explain away or justify our sin, but ultimately, we know in our heart that what we are doing is wrong, but we do it anyway. Because sin separates us from God, this causes inner turmoil resulting in severe negative emotions.

After the couple had their first serving of fruit, their eyes were opened to knowledge and moral discernment. They saw that they were naked and for the first time felt ashamed. Why did they feel shame? They were alone in the garden, no one was looking. They knew they disobeyed God's moral standards and disappointed God, this caused their guilt and shame—the root problem – pride. Shame is a negative emotion. They wanted to be like God, they placed their pride above God's will. Shame - the first negative emotion on earth. Shame keeps us oppressed. They both covered themselves with fig leaves to hide their shame.

One day God came down to the garden. Both Adam and Eve hid from God. Why would they think they could hide from God? But they knew they had sinned and were filled with guilt. God knew what had happened but still asked if they ate from the forbidden tree. Adam said, "The woman whom you gave to be with me, she gave me fruit of the tree, and I ate." Does this sound familiar? We all tend to blame others to mitigate our responsibility for our bad decisions. Adam blamed Eve, and even implicated God in a conspiracy against him saying that God gave him the girl – he didn't want her. God turned to Eve and said, "What is this that you have done?" Eve said, "The serpent deceived me, and I ate." She blamed the serpent.

All behavior has consequences, the discipline for their sin was that God cursed the serpent by forcing him to stay on his belly and eat dust – a symbol of humiliation. God cursed Satan by making him an enemy of those in the family of God. God condemned women to suffer pain in childbirth. This seems to indicate that God's original plan was that childbirth was painless. Secondly, God made it so that the relationship between women and their husbands would be stormy. Women were intended to be man's companion – in marriage, one flesh. A woman's desire is to control her husband, but God put man as the head of the family, Ephesians 5:23-24 says,

"Wives, submit to your own husbands, as to the LORD. For the husband is the head of the wife even as Christ is the head of the church, his body, and is himself its Savior. Now as the church submits to Christ, so also wives should submit in everything to their husbands."

This is one of the most difficult scriptures to follow. So, the rule of love and marriage founded in paradise is replaced by struggle and domination -- a result of the fall.

Adam took the brunt of God's wrath. God blamed Adam, he commanded Adam not to eat of the tree. Adam was responsible for telling Eve. Adam did not accept responsibility for what he had done. God cursed the ground of the earth. Humans would now have a difficult time working the ground for food. This is why most of us have a difficult time making a living. We go through life hating our jobs, never being satisfied in our work.

God banished the couple from paradise forcing them out into the cursed world. God placed angels at the entrances to the garden to prevent anyone from entering. Lastly, God allowed death by separating them from the Tree of Life. Instead of living eternity in the garden, humans would now die. The tree of life returns when we go to heaven, In the Book of Revelation, John describes the new heaven,

"On each side of the river was the tree of life, which bears fruit twelve times a year, once each month; and its leaves are for the healing of the nations." --Revelation 22:2

Their sin separated them from God – spiritual death and banishment from the garden removed them from the Tree of Life – causing eventual physical death. No more walks in the garden with God, no more eternal life with God. Spiritual death is the worst punishment one can receive.

Because of the couple's sin, God instituted the first animal sacrifice to "cover" their sins. The penalty for sin is death, "…sin came into the world through one man, and death through sin, and so death spread to all men because all sinned" (Romans 5:12). Violations of God's moral standard called for a death penalty, "For the wages of sin is death…" (Romans 6:23), and without the shedding of blood there is no forgiveness of sins" (Hebrews 9:22), this is the gospel. In the garden, God killed an animal in order to clothe the couple, to cover their sins. This was the first death on earth. Some theologians suggest the animal was a lamb, but the bible does not say. The shedding of animal blood merely covered their sin. This was the forerunner to Jesus' work on the cross that provided forgiveness to all past, present, and future. This animal sacrifice restored the relationship between Adam and Eve, and God. Even though we will always be forgiven if requested, there are always consequences to our actions.

The ramifications of Adam's sin affected all his future descendants – all the human race. Each person born into this world would no longer be guaranteed provision from the garden, work would now be difficult, life would be hard; our years limited, and even worse, we are all born spiritually dead – separated from God.

The fall brought sin into a perfect world. Our behavior has implications. What we do – good or bad affects others. Adam's sin infected the entire human race with sin (Romans 5:12-21). Every person born is born separated from God because of this imputed sin. The only remedy is to make Jesus your Lord and Savior.

Lastly, since the fall, the authority over the earth has been transferred to Satan. God originally gave authority to humans to control the earth and everything on it. But Adam's sin gave away that authority. Satan is now the god of this world (2 Corinthians 4:4). This is why sin is so dangerous, it gives authority to Satan to oppress us. Sin can devastate one's life, Adam's sin caused a ripple effect that infected all his descendants, including you and me. We must understand that Satan is real and that he does not have your best interest in mind.

CHAPTER FOUR
SATAN'S PLAN

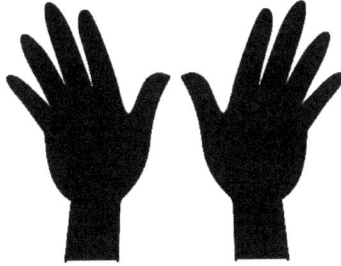

"Be sober-minded; be watchful. Your adversary the devil prowls around like a roaring lion, seeking someone to devour." --1 Peter 5:8

Satan hates God and His followers. Satan in Hebrew means "adversary." His mission is to stop God's goal of salvation to all people and prevent the Kingdom of God from coming. He uses many different strategies to complete his mission, mostly lies and deception to oppress his targets, but he is not above using any destructive activity to cause people to turn away from God and destroy themselves. This is especially true for believers. Why believers? Because non-believers already belong to Satan, no need to expend energy on them.

The Book of Job chapters one and two teach that Satan needs God's permission to inflict pain on anyone. He can influence and oppress people at his will, however, if his intent is to do harm to someone, he needs God's approval. Demons have limited power under God's authority. God is in charge, nothing occurs in life without God's approval. Once this is understood, Christians only need to be aware of their behavior

It is important to understand that as you grow in Christ on your way to spiritual maturity, and grow closer to God, Satan and his demons will step up their harassment of you – attack you. This is bitter-sweet because as you walk in the Holy Spirit, you are fulfilling God's will, when you are in His will, you are producing good fruit (doing good things). Satan does not want you to be a good example of a Christian, he wants you to be a bad witness. Jesus wants us to be a positive light in this dark world, Jesus said in Matthew 5:14-16 says,

> "You are the light of the world. A city set on a hill cannot be hidden. Nor do people light a lamp and put it under a basket, but on a stand, and it gives light to all in the house. In the same way, let your light shine before others, so that they may see your good works and give glory to your Father who is in heaven."

Satan can see that you are that light, but he wants to extinguish the light by influencing you to act like non-believers.

The good news is through Jesus' work on the cross we have authority over Satan and his demons – we have victory over evil. It is our position in Christ that Satan has been defeated. Romans 6:5-7, 11, 14 says,

"For if we have been united with Him [Jesus] in a death like His, we shall certainly be united with Him in a resurrection like His. We know that our old self was crucified with Him in order that the body of sin might be brought to nothing, so that we would no longer be enslaved to sin. For one who has died has been set free from sin."

"So, you also must consider yourselves dead to sin and alive to God in Christ Jesus." v. 11

"For sin will have no dominion over you, since you are not under law but under grace." v. 14

And Colossians 2:15 adds,

"He [Jesus] disarmed the rulers and authorities and put them to open shame, by triumphing over them in Him."

Luke tells us about a time Jesus sent out His 72 disciples to go out into the country to preach and teach the gospel. Before they set out, Jesus gave them authority over evil spirits and illness. When the 72 returned, they were amazed that they were able to heal people and cast out evil spirits in Jesus' name. As a Christian, we possess that same authority as the 72, authority over evil. You are no longer a slave to sin. Satan has no power over you – unless you allow it.

Not all things that are evil are of Satan. Since the fall, humans are born in sin, we have been our worst enemy. The Apostle Paul in his letter to the church in Rome reminds the Christians in Rome that all people are sinners, he said,

> "None is righteous [without sin], no, not one; no one understands; no one seeks for God. All have turned aside; together they have become worthless; no one does good, not even one. Their throat is an open grave; they use their tongues to deceive. The venom of asps [deadly Egyptian Viper] is under their lips. Their mouth is full of curses and bitterness. Their feet are swift to shed blood; in their paths are ruin and misery, and the way of peace they have not known. There is no fear of God before their eyes." -- Romans 3:10-18

We like to lie, cheat, steal, tear down others, we curse others, and promote violence. We do not know how-to live-in peace. This is evidenced by man's constant will to start wars over selfish motives. Things have not changed in thousands of years. No one seeks God – no one. In the Old Testament God said, "The LORD saw that the wickedness of man was great in the earth, and that every intention of the thoughts of his heart was only evil continually" (Genesis 6:5). And the prophet Jeremiah records what God told him, "The heart is deceitful above all things, and desperately sick; who can understand it?" (v. 17:9).

In Mark chapter seven, we read about when the high priests saw that Jesus and His disciples did not follow Jewish traditions like washing hands prior to meals. Jesus said,

> "And He [Jesus] said to them [high priests], 'Then are you also without understanding? Do you not see that whatever goes into a person from outside cannot defile him, since it enters not his heart but his stomach, and is expelled?' And He said, 'What comes out of a person is

what defiles him. For from within, out of the heart of man, come evil thoughts, sexual immorality, theft, murder, adultery, coveting, wickedness, deceit, sensuality, envy, slander, pride, foolishness. All these evil things come from within, and they defile a person'" -- Mark 7:18-23

Jesus is telling them that sin begins in the heart. The Jewish elite practiced ritual washing, believing that they would be spiritually clean. But Jesus said cleansing the outside does not make you clean, nor does what you eat (referring to rules against eating pork) because sin comes from the inside. Jesus was saying a rebellious heart makes you unclean. We need to spiritually cleanse by confession and repentance.

It is not only sin that opens the door for Satan's oppression. Participating in occult activities invites evil spirits into our lives. We see on television and hear about fortune-tellers, mediums, and psychics who can tell you accurate information about your past and predict your future. Some of these spiritualists are con artists. There are some who do connect with the spiritual world, but these are evil spirits. God forbids the use of others to do His job. Deuteronomy 18:10-12 says,

"There shall not be found among you anyone who burns his son or his daughter as an offering, anyone who practices divination or tells fortunes or interprets omens, or a sorcerer or a charmer or a medium or a necromancer or one who inquires of the dead, for whoever does these things is an abomination to the LORD. And because of these abominations, the LORD your God is driving them out before you."

These psychics are often under Satan's influence. They connect with the evil spirit responsible for your oppression, that spirit cannot read your mind but has been watching you since birth. They know everything about you and relay it to the psychic, who then takes credit for knowing all about you. If you have been involved in any occult activity, please confess and renounce your involvement to restore your relationship with God.

Almost everyone believes that they are a good person – better than they really are. We lie to ourselves, not accepting that we have an evil side. People do a very good job of bringing evil into our communities. We cannot blame Satan for all the bad things in this world. Our sinful flesh can give Satan a run for his money. The good news is that we can change our evil hearts by accepting Jesus Christ as our Lord and Savior. The Holy Spirit will change you from the inside out. We will talk more about that later.

CHAPTER FIVE

SIN

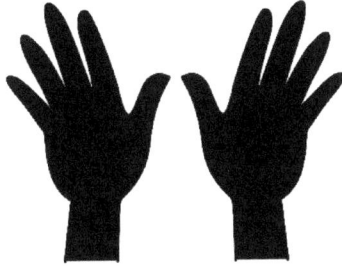

"...There is no health in my bones because of my sin." -
-Psalm 38:3-6

Sin means "missing the mark." Sin is rebellion against God. Sin disrupts our relationship with God, it takes us out of fellowship with Him. Missing the mark suggests that there was a correct mark or target, and we missed it. The target would be doing God's will or simply doing the right thing. The Apostle John defines sin as "lawlessness" (1 John 3:4). Sin can also be defined as a lack of conformity to God's moral standards.

Every person on earth is a descendant of Adam and Eve, Adam's sin corrupted all his descendants. We all have the tendency to lie, cheat, and steal. If you say that you have never committed any of these sins, you lie. Sin is engrained in us from birth. If you are a parent, you know that when you tell your child to not do something, they will do it.

We also see this pattern in how children play games. They always cheat. I lost a lot of games of checkers until I realized they cheat. These are all symptoms of a fallen world. It is our nature; we all have it. We were created with the knowledge of right and wrong, it's written on our hearts. Children know when they push another child down that it is wrong to hurt others, we also know that helping others is good. But what do we do most of? Self-serving activities!

We often choose to sin and ignore our conscience. Everyone has a sinful nature, even the Apostle Paul wrestled with sin, and he was chosen by God to write a large portion of the New Testament and to spread the gospel. Romans 7:15-20 says,

> "For I [Paul] do not understand my own actions. For I do not do what I want, but I do the very thing I hate… So it is no longer I that do it, but the sin that dwells within me. For I know that nothing good dwells in me, that is, in my flesh. For I have the desire to do what is right, but not the ability to carry it out. For I do not do the good I want but the evil I do not want, it is no longer I who do it, but the sin that dwells within me."

This is a difficult concept to grab a hold of, we all believe ourselves to be good people. But our beliefs are according to what the world believes is "good." Inside us, we have the capacity to do evil. In order to determine where our relationship with God is we must examine our life. Is there any unrepented sin? Are you walking in alignment with God? Do you need to forgive someone? Do you need to ask forgiveness from someone? Or, are you loving one another as Jesus commands? If you are in habitual sin, you could be subject to illness and disease. Repentance is the only cure for sin. Jesus' brother James, confirms this teaching by saying that when you are sick, go to the church and confess your sins to each other, pray for one another so you will be healed (James 5:13-16).

We also must understand the spiritual laws and principles relating to sin. The bible teaches that everything we do results in a consequence – for good behavior – blessings and for bad behavior -- discipline. Galatians 6:7-8 says,

> "Do not be deceived: God is not mocked, for whatever one sows, that will he also reap. For the one who sows to his own flesh will from the flesh reap corruption, but the one who sows to the Spirit will from the Spirit reap eternal life. And let us not grow weary of doing good, for in due season we will reap, if we do not give up."

Sowing and reaping are agricultural terms that the people in biblical times would have understood. Sowing means to plant seed or set something in motion. Reaping means to gather, to obtain something, or to obtain the results of what you set in motion. If you do something good (in God's will) you will receive good in return. If you commit a sinful act (against God's will) you will receive bad in return. We often do not receive your returns immediately; it could take months or even years to reap your returns.

An associated principle is called the "Law of Increase." God told the prophet Hosea, "For they [Israel] sow to the wind, and they reap the whirlwind" This law is "cause-and-effect." Do good and more good will come to you. Do bad and more bad will come to you. In another letter to the church in Corinth, Paul teaches the importance of giving generously to those in need. Paul says,

> "The point is this, whoever sows sparingly will also reap sparingly, and whoever sows bountifully, will reap bountifully." --2 Corinthians 9:6

And Jesus taught His disciples,

> "Pay attention to what you hear, with the measure you use, it will be measured to you, and still more will be added to you." --Mark 4:24-25

We also must understand a life principle, the Law of Diminishing Returns. When you sin, the Holy Spirit will convict you of your sin telling you that you did something wrong. Everyone knows right from wrong. God wrote right and wrong in our hearts. The problem is that we normally don't listen to our conscience/heart.

The first time you commit a sin, the Holy Spirit will tell you that you did something out of God's will. God talks to you through your conscience to tell you that you went against God's moral standards and need to repent for that wrong. If you ignore that little voice of your conscience and repeat that same sin – you "sear your conscience." The definition of *sear* is to make withered and dried up. As you continue in this sin, your conscience bothers you less and less. Your conscience begins to wither and die. Some may say you build a callus over your conscience – your sense of right and wrong. Eventually, your conscience will stop warning you. You can then sin with impunity of your conscience. Soon you justify your behavior, no matter how bad. This same process applies to Christians. If you continue in your habitual sin, you grieve the Holy Spirit, who will soon give you over to your sin.

The law of diminishing returns can also be compared to drug/alcohol tolerance. The first time you use a legal or illegal drug or drink alcohol, its impact on the body is powerful. It only takes a small amount to achieve the desired effect. The more often you use the substance, the more your body builds a tolerance to the substance. You then have to use larger amounts of the substance to obtain the desired effect. After long-term use, your body has built a tolerance so that the drug will no longer get you "high." The body then needs the substance just to "feel normal." This is addiction, you're now a slave to that substance. It is the same with sin.

When our conscience has been seared, we remain in habitual sin, the sin then controls us (John 8:35). The sin controls our day-to-day behavior, as well as all our relationships with others. Sin is nothing more than a person's attempt to find peace and meaning.

Since the fall, we have all been born with a hole in our heart. We know it's there because we sense that something is missing. We seek out ways to fill that hole, we try money, power/control, substances, gambling, or sex, just to name a few. Humans tend to seek for meaning, purpose, and joy in their lives. We believe that if we just had the newest Corvette, a facelift, or a Rolex watch, people would love and respect us. These things we seek out become idols in our lives. We place them above our relationship with God. Nothing will fill that hole in your heart because it is God-shaped. It is only God that can make your heart whole. When you allow God to fill that void, peace, and joy are the results.

The only way to prevent the law of increase from becoming dominant in your life is to make Jesus Christ your Lord and Savior. When you do, God's Holy Spirit lives in your heart and renews your conscience. Listening and following the Holy Spirit's guidance prevents you from becoming a slave to your sin. When you do sin, and you will, you will hear God's voice telling you to stop. Listen to the voice, stop! Confess and repent, then pray for God's strength to help you overcome the temptation.

What if we sin? First, let me say —we all sin, and always will, so do not stress. All you have to do to restore fellowship with God is to acknowledge your sin and repent and your relationship is restored.

CHAPTER SIX

EVIL

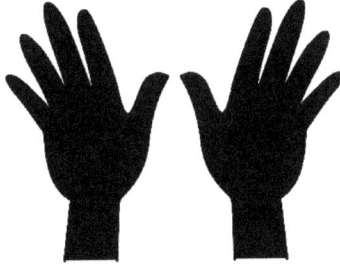

"For we know that the law is spiritual, but I am of the flesh, sold under sin. For I [Paul] do not understand my own actions. For I do not do what I want, but I do the very thing I hate. Now if I do what I do not want I agree with the law, that it is good. So now it is no longer I who do it, but sin that dwells within me. For I know that nothing good dwells in me, that is, in my flesh. For I have the desire to do what is right, but not the ability to carry it out. For I do not do the good I want, but the evil I do not want is what I keep on doing. Now if I do what I do not want, it is no longer I who do it, but sin that dwells within me. So I find it to be law that when I want to do right, evil lies close at hand." --Romans 7:14-21

For over 3,000 years, people have been asking the question, why do evil people seem to prosper? This bothered the prophet Jeremiah who asked God, "Righteous are you, O LORD, when I complain to you; yet I would plead my case before you. Why does the way of the wicked prosper? Why do all who are treacherous thrive?" (Jeremiah 12:1).

Since the fall, the world is full of evil. What is *evil*? Evil can be defined as offensive sinful, or wicked. Where did evil come from? Did God create evil? Evil is not a person, place, or thing, it is not a substance. Evil is a character trait, a *belief*, an *attitude* that manifests in *behavior*. So, the answer is that God did not create evil. However, God created heavenly beings and the human race; He created them with the freedom of choice, and all too often His created beings choose evil.

God hates evil. If God did not create evil and He hates it, why does He allow evil to exist? This is a difficult question to answer. God is all-powerful, He can do anything. He is a loving God; He doesn't wish to see any of His creations suffer. In order to eradicate evil, He would have to take away our freedom of choice. We would be like robots programmed to love God and do good. No one would like that.

Let's look at the first sin in the universe. God created angels with freedom of choice. The first sin ever committed was by a high-ranking beautiful angel named Lucifer. The Bible says Lucifer was one of God's greatest cherubim. Cherubim were created to guard the holiness of God. Lucifer became corrupted by pride. Lucifer knew he was beautiful and powerful. The prophet Isaiah describes Lucifer's fall in Isaiah 14:12-15,

> "How you [Lucifer] are fallen from heaven... You said in your heart, 'I will ascend to heaven; above the stars of God I will set my throne on high; I will sit on the mount

of assembly in the far reaches of the north; I will ascend above the heights of the clouds; I will make myself like the Most High [God].' But you are brought down to Sheol [refers to the grave or the abode of the dead], to the far reaches of the pit."

Lucifer's pride swelled. He wanted to place himself above God's throne. Pride is a sin, sin has consequences. God banished Lucifer from heaven to earth. Lucifer is now called Satan, which means "adversary or accuser." One-third of all the angels in heaven chose to follow Lucifer to earth. Those angels are now called fallen angels, evil spirits, or demons. They do Satan's work. The Bible does not tell us when this occurred in relation to the creation of humans. But common sense would lead us to believe that this occurred after the creation of the earth and before Adam's creation. Satan hates God and those who follow Him. Satan's goal is to prevent as many people as possible from knowing God.

After the fall, Adam gave dominion of the earth to Satan. Satan is now "the god of this world" (2 Corinthians 4:4). Satan blocks the mind of non-believers so that when they hear the gospel, they will not understand it, then reject it (2 Corinthians 4:3-4). Satan rules the systems of the world that goes against God's moral standards.

Jesus commands us to make disciples of all the world. In relation to Christians, Satan's mission is to render us ineffective in our testimony discipleship by preventing us from maturing spiritually. This is done through *temptation*. He tempts us with the "pleasures of the world." Satan is not all-knowing, all-powerful, nor is he in all places at the same time. He cannot read our thoughts, but He is an expert in human behavior. Satan and his demons have been watching human beings for thousands of years. They watch you and make notes on your likes, dislikes, and secret fetishes – all to be used against you as a temptation when the time is right. He cannot read your thoughts, but he listens to your conversations, he hears who we dislike, he sees what websites we go to, and he patiently waits for a time to use this all against you.

The Bible tells us that Satan goes back and forth on the earth looking for people to devour. His goal is to get you to sin because he knows that sin separates you from God. When your relationship with God is disrupted, he plays on your guilt and fear, which causes your negative emotions. He will lie to you telling you that you are no good, that God doesn't love you, and that He will never forgive you. He tries to keep you in emotional pain and tells us that it is God's fault. He exploits our desires and dreams. The longer we stay in pain, the further away from God we get. Mission accomplished!

Sin is the *root cause* of our separation from God. The result of separation is emotional pain, sin cause chaos in our spirit. The cure is to restore your relationship with God.

It was poor selfish choices that brought sin into the world—First Lucifer, then Adam. God wants you to love Him by your own choice. He will not force you to follow Him. But since the fall, humans have chosen to do their own thing, be their own god.

The story of the great flood in Genesis chapters six through nine tells how God tried to put an end to evil by killing everyone on earth except for eight people. The Bible says the population of the earth multiplied greatly due to the longevity of life at that time. Some people lived up to 900 years. The people on Earth were evil. Scriptures say that God saw that man's heart and intentions were evil. God said He was sorry that He had created humans. In order to cleanse the earth, God decided to end the evil by killing everything on earth except for eight people and two of each animal in order to cleanse the land. He chose a man named Noah and his family to repopulate the earth. Genesis 6:11-13 says,

> "Now the earth was corrupt in God's sight, and the earth was filled with violence. And God saw the earth, and behold, it was corrupt, for all flesh had corrupted their way on the earth. And God said to Noah, 'I have determined to make an end of all flesh, for the earth is filled with violence through them. Behold, I will destroy them with the earth.'"

God told Noah to build an ark that was big enough to carry Noah, his family, and all the animals. Noah built the ship and when the time was right, God brought rain, and water flooded the entire earth. The Bible says that the water level was twenty feet above the tallest mountain. Every living thing on earth died. Once everything had died, God ordered the flood waters to recede. When the waters receded and Noah, his family, and the animals were safe, God said,

"Then Noah built an altar to the LORD and took some of every clean animal and some of every clean bird and offered burnt offerings on the altar. And when the LORD smelled the pleasing aroma, the LORD said in his heart, 'I will never again curse the ground because of man, for the intention of man's heart is evil from his youth. Neither will I ever again strike down every living creature as I have done.'" --Genesis 8:20-21

God blessed Noah and his family and told them to be fruitful and multiply. At this point, God gave the people all living things to eat with one limitation, not to eat flesh with the blood still in it; it must be cooked. This is because blood is life. And, God instituted a new law – if someone kills another person, their punishment will be death. Every person is made in God's image, therefore, killing a person shows contempt for God. God now also limited the length of human life in future generations to 120 years.

God tried to put an end to evil, but our flesh is inherently evil. Evil and pride soon returned to rule the earth. Since the fall, evil has ruled on the earth. Evil manifests itself in violence, racism, hunger, hate, disease, oppression, and many other ways. God did not create evil, it originated from an angel's freedom of choice to follow his creator or to be his own god. Adam and Eve made the same poor choice. Now every person on earth is born with this sinful nature and is spiritually dead. It is only through faith and trust in Jesus Christ that we are reborn and regenerated, being spiritually alive.

As Christians, we must accept that evil exists. Jesus taught that good and evil co-exist on earth. Matthew 13:24-30 describes when Jesus told a parable of a farmer (represents Jesus) sowing seeds. The farmer planted wheat seeds (represents Christians) in His field (the earth). At night, the enemy (Satan) went into the field and planted weeds (evil people) next to the wheat. As the wheat grew up, the weeds surrounded the wheat. The workers (represents angels) of the field told the farmer about the weeds.

The workers wanted to pull out all the weeds (remove the evil people). The farmer told the workers to leave the weeds in the ground because some wheat may accidentally be uprooted as the weeds are pulled. The farmer insisted that the weeds grow up together with the wheat to protect every bit of wheat. At harvest time, when the wheat and weeds are pulled, the weeds are burned in the fire (hell), referring to the second coming of Jesus when He will judge non-believers, Jesus said,

> "Just as the weeds are gathered and burned with fire, so will it be at the end of the age. The Son of Man will send His angels, and they will gather out of His kingdom all causes of sin and all law-breakers, and throw them into the fiery furnace. In that place there will be weeping and gnashing of teeth. Then the righteous will shine like the sun in the kingdom of their Father." --Matthew 13:40-43

Jesus is telling us that in this world, there is good and evil, Jesus will remove the evil at His second coming. Proverbs 11:21 says, "Be assured an evil person will not go unpunished, but the offspring of the righteous will be delivered." Between now and then, we must trust in God in order to persevere in these evil times.

God created people to have the freedom to choose their own route in life – many people choose the sinful way. Jesus said,

> "Do for others what you want them to do for you: this is the meaning of the Law of Moses and of the teachings of the prophets. Go in through the narrow gate, because the gate to hell is wide and the road that leads to it is easy, and there are many who travel it. But the gate to life is narrow and the way that leads to it is hard, and there are few people who find it." --Matthew 7:12-14

Jesus is saying that not many people will choose to follow God, they will choose the way of the world. Choosing a sinful life leads to judgment, choosing to follow God will bring eternal life. Sinful living brings consequences. Sometimes those consequences affect other people—innocent people. We can see this every day in the news: drunk drivers harm innocent people, chemical companies try to save money by dumping hazardous chemicals in streams and emotionally disturbed people shoot into crowds of innocent people with the intent to kill. Jesus warns us that there will be difficult times in life due to the presence of evil, and innocent people will be victimized.

The question is: Why doesn't God intervene? The answer is that God cannot interfere with people's freedom of choice. God is not indifferent to pain and suffering. The first two chapters of the Book of Job teach that God places limits on Satan's plans. God knows how much we can take and how much pain to inflict to obtain the desired results. God is able to restrain Satan, bring us out of our pain, and fulfill His plan for our lives.

God gets intimately involved post-event. He uses the evil that Satan causes to bring forth something positive for believers and the kingdom of God (Romans 8:28). He changes what Satan meant for evil to work for the good.

We must not place too much emphasis on Satan. Through Jesus' death and resurrection, Satan is defeated. Satan is now subject to the authority of Jesus. Satan only poses a threat to us if we allow him. Satan is evil, but humans can be just as evil on their own.

The flesh has great power over us. Selfish desires appear to be our default setting. God has written right and wrong in our hearts. We instinctively know the right thing to do, but for some reason, our flesh influences us to not do the right thing.

God told the prophet, Jeremiah,

> "Thus says the LORD: 'Cursed is the man who trusts in man and makes flesh his strength, whose heart turns away from the LORD.'" --Job 17:5

The term "flesh" refers to our own desires. Paul talks about the flesh in his letter to the Christians in Galatia,

> "But I say, walk by the Spirit, and you will not gratify the desires of the flesh. For the desires of the flesh are against the Spirit, and the desires of the Spirit are against the flesh, for these are opposed to each other, to keep you

from doing the things you want to do. But if you are led by the Spirit, you are not under the law. Now the works of the flesh are evident: sexual immorality, impurity, sensuality, idolatry, sorcery, enmity, strife, jealousy, fits of anger, rivalries, dissensions, divisions, envy, drunkenness, orgies, and things like these. I warn you, as I warned you before, that those who do such things will not inherit the kingdom of God." -- Galatians 5:16-21

Jesus' brother James 4:17 says that if we know the right thing to do but do not do it, it's a sin. Every human being is tempted by their flesh. Paul experienced the same temptations 2000 years ago, he wrote,

"For I do not understand my own actions. For I do not do what I want, but I do the very thing I hate. Now if I do what I do not want, I agree with the law, that it is good. So now it is no longer I who do it, but sin that dwells within me. For I know that nothing good dwells in me, that is, in my flesh. For I have the desire to do what is right, but not the ability to carry it out. For I do not do the good I want, but the evil I do not want is what I keep on doing. Now if I do what I do not want, it is no longer I who do it, but sin that dwells within me." -- Romans 7:15-20

Paul was possibly the greatest apostle and he went through the same temptations as we do today. This makes me feel better.

Why does our flesh have so much power over us? Throughout our lives we conform to this world. Since our birth, we have been influenced by societal norms. We learn to look out for number one – ourselves! We learn to lie or blame others to get out of trouble, we learn survival of the fittest. If you want it – take it! These beliefs become strongholds and dictate our behavior. Influencers include parents, teachers, television, movies, friends, and many more. Jesus warns us to not be conformed to this world, don't get comfortable.

How do we overcome these strongholds so that we can resist temptations? Make Jesus Christ your Lord and Savior. When you are born again, God's Holy Spirit lives in your heart. The power of the Holy Spirit is incredible. John said, "For everyone who has been born of God overcomes the world. And this is the victory that has overcome the world—our faith" (1 John 5:4).

If evil is our default setting and God will not withdraw our freedom of choice, what is God's role? I believe it is God's role to mitigate the damage of our poor choices. God ensures that our pain will always have a reason – a meaning. Some reasons include: bringing us closer to Him, refining us, humbling us, disciplining us, and to fulfill His plan. It is difficult to accept, but all these things work for our good. It's all about perspective. When we look at our pain through the eyes of God, we see that God works all things for the good of God's kingdom (Romans 8:28-29).

We have two adversaries: Satan and our flesh. Under our own power, defeating both is impossible. But all things are possible in Christ. There will be trials in our lives, but with the power of the Holy Spirit, we will overcome them.

God will work the evil that you went through for your good. Your pain has a purpose, and that purpose is to be conformed not to the world, but into the image of the Son of God.

CHAPTER SEVEN

SEVEN REASONS WHY GOD ALLOWS SUFFERING IN OUR LIVES:

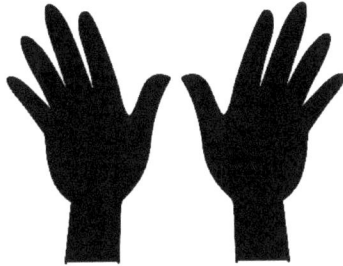

1. TO FULFILL GOD'S PLAN

"Many are the plans in the mind of a man, but it is the purpose of the LORD that will stand." --Proverbs 19:21

God is all-powerful, all-knowing, at in every place at the same time. God has a plan and purpose for every person on this earth – both believers and non-believers. It is God that executes that plan by directing all things in order that His will is accomplished. The term for this is providence. God will ensure that His *will* – will be done.

God has two types of will. The first is called God's *revealed will,* which dictates His moral standards, and how we conduct ourselves. God's moral and ethical standards are revealed in His commandments. God has revealed these standards to us through the bible and the Holy Spirit. For example, we know it is God's will for believers to be conformed to the image of His son (Romans 8:29) because He has revealed it to us.

God also has a *secret will*. An example of His secret will is the story of Jonah. God told the prophet Jonah to go to the city of Nineveh and preach repentance; if the people did not repent, God would destroy the city. The people of Nineveh were very cruel to the Jewish people – they hated each other. Jonah did not want his enemy to be saved – he wanted them to be destroyed. But God had a different plan. We know it is God's *revealed* will that says,

> "For God so loved the world, that He gave his only Son, that whoever believes in Him should not perish but have eternal life. For God did not send his Son into the world to condemn the world, but in order that the world might be saved through Him." --John 3:16-17

God wants all people saved. Jonah ran in the opposite direction; he did not want his enemy to be saved. God brought adversity into Jonah's life which forced him to do God's will; Jonah went to Nineveh and preached repentance. The city of 600,000 was saved. It is God's *revealed will* to save all people. It was His *secret will* that specifically sent Jonah to the city of Nineveh to be saved. This story is also a great example of following God's calling. God's will – will be done. It can be done the easy way or the hard way – you choose.

God chooses all types of people to orchestrate His will. There are many examples in the bible of God using people who are down and out, as well as people who are devout. The important point to understand is that God uses people to fulfill His will. God is a spirit. He has no physical body. His followers are His hands, feet, and voice on earth to accomplish His work. It is an honor to be chosen by God, but some of the time, God's chosen people will be forced to endure some pain or suffering during the fulfillment of that plan. An often-used example is the story of Joseph in Genesis chapters 37-50.

Joseph is a descendant of Abraham, who is the father of Israel and the first Hebrew. God chose Abraham to institute the Nation of Israel. Upon Abraham's death, his son Isaac led Israel. When Isaac died, his son Jacob led Israel. God changed Jacob's name to Israel. Israel had twelve children who later became the twelve tribes of Israel, he was a rich man and had many herds of livestock.

Joseph was Israel's eleventh son. Israel loved Joseph more than all his other sons and made no effort to conceal that fact. Israel had a special coat made for Joseph. This caused Joseph's brothers to become jealous, and they hated him for being the favorite.

When Joseph was seventeen years old, he had dreams that one day his family would bow down to him. During those times the eldest son was revered, and the youngest served to the oldest. Jacob and his sons were outraged that Joseph would be so prideful and brag about his dream. His brothers hated Joseph even more.

One day Joseph's brothers were out taking care of the animals. Israel asked Joseph to go and check on them. When the brothers were about twenty miles away, they saw Joseph approaching, they agreed to kill him and hide his body in a cistern. A cistern is a deep pit in the ground used to store water for the people and animals to drink. They planned to kill Joseph and put animal blood on his unique coat and tell their father that an animal killed and ate Joseph. One of the brothers, Reuben, did not want to kill Joseph, he suggested that they just leave Joseph in the cistern. Reuben planned to rescue Joseph later.

When Joseph arrived, the brothers took his coat and threw him into a dry cistern. The brothers then sat down and had lunch. As they ate, the men saw a caravan of merchandise traders approaching. They sold Joseph as a slave for twenty shekels. These Midianite traders later sold Joseph to the Ishmaelites, who took him to Egypt and sold him to a high-ranking government official.

Joseph was most likely tied up and forced to walk behind the caravan in the blazing heat. He probably had little to no food or water for the 200 miles to Egypt. He felt betrayed and scared not knowing if he was going to live or die. The brothers tore Joseph's coat and dipped it in animal blood. They told Israel that an animal had attacked and killed Joseph. Israel cried out in grief and mourned for a long time. No one could console him.

Potiphar, the pharaoh's captain of the guard, purchased Joseph to work in his home. Joseph was a slave, but the scriptures say that God was with Joseph and blessed all he did. Potiphar promoted Joseph to be in charge of all his household. With Joseph in charge, Potiphar had no worries – he trusted Joseph.

Joseph was a very handsome and fit young man. Potiphar's wife tried many times to seduce Joseph. He always refused, not wanting to violate Potiphar's trust. Joseph said, "How can I do this great wickedness and sin against God?" One day he was working in the house, and no others were around. Potiphar's wife grabbed him by the robe, saying, "Lie with me." He ran out of the house; she tore his robe off him as he fled. She was angry that he rejected her and yelled for help from the guards. She told the guards that Joseph tried to rape her, but she fought him off. When Potiphar heard this, he became angry and had Joseph arrested and thrown in jail. By this time, Joseph had been enslaved in Egypt for two or three years. He missed his family – especially his father. He was alone in a foreign land, falsely accused of rape, and sitting in prison for who knows how long. I bet he cried out to God many times, asking, "Why?"

Even in prison, God was with Joseph, giving him favor in all he did. The warden saw God's favor was with Joseph and placed him in charge of the entire prison and over every inmate. The warden trusted Joseph and did not worry about any issue in the prison. Whatever Joseph did, God made it successful. But Joseph was still sad and lonely, missing his family. He may have even doubted God's love at times, just as we do during trials in our lives.

One day the pharaoh's cupbearer, who served drinks, and the pharaoh's baker committed an unknown crime, and both were placed in prison. Joseph was appointed to attend to them. A few years later, both the cupbearer and baker had strange dreams. They asked Joseph if he could interpret the dreams. Joseph told them that it is only God that interprets a person's dream. The pair told Joseph the details of their dreams. God revealed the interpretation of the dreams to Joseph.

The cupbearer's dream was interpreted to mean that in three days, the pharaoh would restore him to his cupbearer's job. Joseph asked the cupbearer to remember him when he returned to serve the pharaoh and to tell him of Joseph's innocence. God revealed the baker's dream to mean that in three days, the pharaoh would order his execution by hanging.

Three days later, it was the pharaoh's birthday, he restored the cupbearer's job and ordered the baker executed. The cupbearer returned to the pharaoh but did not tell him about Joseph. I imagine that Joseph became excited that the cupbearer was going to get him out of prison. Joseph was innocent but remained in prison for several years – his release did not come. This loneliness would have caused frustration and depression. Although the text doesn't talk about Joseph's emotional condition, he must have been disappointed.

A few weeks later, the pharaoh had some disturbing dreams. He sent for magicians and wise men to interpret the dreams. No one could interpret the pharaoh's dream. The cupbearer remembered Joseph and told him that there was a man named Joseph in prison who interpreted dreams. The pharaoh ordered that Joseph be brought to the palace.

It had been thirteen years since Joseph was brought to Egypt. He had spent the last ten years in prison. The pharaoh's servants went to get Joseph out of prison and cleaned, shaved and dressed

Joseph. They brought him to the palace to meet the pharaoh. The pharaoh asked Joseph if he could interpret dreams. Joseph said, "It is not in me, God will give pharaoh a favorable answer." The pharaoh told Joseph his dreams. God revealed the meaning of the dreams to Joseph. The dream was that there were to be seven years of prosperity in Egypt and a warning of a seven-year famine at the end of the seven years. God told Joseph that this was going to begin very soon and that the pharaoh needed to select a discerning and wise man to prepare and plan to allow Egypt to survive the years of famine. Joseph suggested that Egypt begin storing a percentage of the food that is harvested during the first seven years. All food and grain should be stored in storage buildings all across Egypt. The stored food would then be rationed out during the years of famine.

Joseph's plan pleased the pharaoh. Pharaoh said, "Can we find a man like this, in whom is the Spirit of God?" – Genesis 41:38.

The pharaoh said to Joseph,

> "Since God has shown you all this, there is none so discerning and wise as you are. You shall be over my house, and all my people shall order themselves as you command. Only as regards the throne will I be greater than you." –Genesis 41:39-41

Pharaoh responded,

> "…I have set you over all the land of Egypt…" "I am Pharaoh, and without your consent no one shall lift up hand or foot in all the land of Egypt." –Genesis 41:41

The pharaoh dressed Joseph in royal robes and jewelry and gave his daughter to him in marriage, Joseph was thirty years old.

Joseph was sold into slavery when he was seventeen years old. He had been blessed by God his entire life. Even though he was a slave and in prison, God was with him. He may not have felt that he was blessed, but God had a plan and purpose for his life. God's plan was to get him to Egypt, although he was in prison, at the right time, he went to the palace. He went from the prison to the palace and was second in command of the entire country of Egypt. God was working behind the scenes. God's plan was to promote Joseph to this powerful position. Why? Let's see:

During the seven years of prosperity, Joseph stored up huge amounts of food that the bible says could not be counted. During this time, Joseph began a family. He had two sons. He named his first son Manasseh, which means "God made me forget all my hardship and all my father's house." His second son, Ephraim, "For God has made me fruitful in the land of my affliction."

After the seven years of plenty came seven years of famine. This famine affected the entire earth. People from all over the world went to Egypt to buy food and grain. Joseph was in charge of the sales, everyone had to go through him to purchase food.

Joseph's father heard there was food in Egypt. The famine was so severe, he thought they would starve to death. He sent his sons to Egypt to purchase grain for the family. All the boys went to Egypt except for the youngest son Benjamin. Benjamin was Jacob's youngest and favorite son.

When the brothers arrived in Egypt, Joseph recognized them. But they did not recognize Joseph. Joseph spoke harshly to them and accused them of being spies. The brothers denied the accusation and explained that they were twelve brothers, one was dead, and the youngest was at home with his father. Joseph said he did not believe them. Joseph told the brothers he wanted to see the youngest boy to prove they were truthful, they were hesitant. Joseph had them thrown in jail.

After the brothers had been in jail for three days, Joseph told them to leave one brother in jail, and the rest go to their home in Canaan and bring back their youngest brother to verify their story. The brothers talked it over, and Joseph listened. The brothers did not know that Joseph spoke Hebrew because they spoke through an interpreter. The brothers believed that this was God's punishment for them for what they did to Joseph. The brothers agreed to go get Benjamin and return. Joseph kept Simeon in jail and gave the men all the food they could carry on their donkeys. The men paid for the grain; however, Joseph had his servants return the money in the food pouches. The brothers left Egypt for Canaan.

When they came to their first stop, they found their money was returned to their sacks. They were scared because they didn't know how it got there, they said, "What is this God has done to us?" When they got home and told their father what had happened, Israel refused to allow Benjamin to go to Egypt. As the famine continued, the food ran out, and Israel was forced to send his sons, including Benjamin, to Egypt. When they arrived in Egypt, Joseph saw Benjamin and ordered a huge feast for the men. Simeon was released from jail, and they all ate.

Joseph sold the men more grain. He had his servants return the money the same as on their first trip. He also ordered his servant to take Joseph's silver drinking cup and put it in Benjamin's sack. As the men were leaving, Joseph had them stopped and searched. They found the money and the cup; the men were accused of theft and detained. The men were returned to Joseph. Joseph toyed with them for a while threatening to make Benjamin a slave. They begged Joseph not to do this, it would kill their father to lose a second son. Judah offered himself to be a slave to let Benjamin go. Joseph could no longer control himself, he cried out and said, "I am Joseph! Is my father still alive?" The men were frightened because they thought that Joseph would seek revenge for what they did to him. Joseph said,

> "...I am your brother, Joseph, whom you sold into Egypt. And now do not be distressed or angry with yourselves because you sold me here, for God sent me before you to preserve life. For the famine has been in the land these two years, and there are yet five years in which there will be neither plowing nor harvest. And God sent me before you to preserve for you a remnant on earth, and to keep alive for you many survivors. So it was not you who sent me here, but God." --Genesis 45:4-8

Joseph told his brothers to bring their father and all the family and move them to Egypt during the famine. Since the pharaoh respected Joseph, he allowed his family to possess the best plots of land in Egypt. Israel's family moved to Egypt, and God blessed them there, his family numbered seventy when they moved to Egypt. At the time of the exodus, the Israelites multiplied to well over one million.

When Israel died, the brothers were scared that Joseph would seek revenge on them. They went to Joseph and fell down before him, begging for forgiveness. Joseph said,

> "Do not fear, for am I in the place of God? As for you, you meant evil against me, but God meant it for good, to bring it about that many people should be kept alive, as they are today." --Genesis 5:19-20

Joseph forgave and comforted his brothers.

The story of Joseph shows how God's secret will was to save the fledgling nation of Israel. He did this by using Joseph's brother's envy and their propensity for evil to fulfill His ultimate plan. Unfortunately, the plan required Joseph to suffer for many years. This is an important theological principle. The story also provides hope to those who understand this principle. Joseph was betrayed by his brothers, sold into slavery, falsely accused, imprisoned, and betrayed again in prison. But, during all this, the Bible says, "The LORD was with Joseph." God's plan served two purposes. The first, like the flood, the famine may have been intended to discipline someone or a nation(s) on earth; or to bring them to repentance. Secondly, because of the famine, the

Hebrews were brought together in one place in order to form the people into a nation. Joseph said that God sent him out before them to prepare and preserve a remnant of the Hebrew people on earth to ensure their growth and survival. The Hebrew nation began with seventy people, which grew to over one million at the time of the exodus. God predestined Joseph to save the Israelite Nation and Egypt. God used Joseph's brothers, who already harbored hate and evil in their hearts. God knew they would willingly kill Joseph. God ordained the merchant traders to cross their paths at the perfect time. By enacting this plan, Joseph was required to suffer some pain, emotional and physical, but God was always with him, not giving him more pain than he could handle. Some may ask, "Why didn't God choose an easier way?" God could have, but we don't know how many sub-plans God was working on in these two primary plans. Each one of our lives touches many other lives. We will not know how we impacted other lives until we get to heaven. God revealed to Joseph His divine plan for Israel. God used the traders, Potiphar's wife, Potiphar, and the cupbearer all to place him in a position that he needed to be to fulfill the plan.

God allowing people to suffer to fulfill His plan is a difficult concept to comprehend. When we understand it, all our cares and worries go out the window.

My last example is of the most-evil event in human history that was planned and ordained by God. I'm referring to the crucifixion of the Son of God – Jesus Christ. This story is told in Matthew chapters 26-27, Mark chapters 14-15, and Luke chapters 22-23. God not only planned these events, but He was actively involved in the actions and events in it. Every person from the religious elite, Judas, and the Roman soldiers who tortured Jesus and crucified Him had evil intentions in their hearts. God used their evil intentions to fulfill His divine plan. Luke tells us in Acts 2:23,

> "...this Jesus, delivered up according to the definite plan and foreknowledge of God. You [Jews] crucified and killed by the hand of the lawless [evil] men."

And Acts 4:27-28 adds,

> "...for truly in this city there were gathered together against Your [God] holy servant Jesus, whom You anointed, both Herod and Pontius Pilate, along with the Gentiles and the peoples of Israel, to do whatever Your hand and Your plan had predestined to take place."

All the participants in Jesus' crucifixion were predestined by God due to their evil hearts. There can be no blame placed on God. God used men that already had impure hearts, God does not force people to do evil acts against their will. These people already had a propensity to commit evil acts, these are the lawless men that Luke speaks of. God knows the heart of every person; He knows who will and will not commit evil acts. We cannot blame God for the evil actions of a person. James warns us,

> "Let no one say when he is tempted, 'I am being tempted by God,' for God cannot be tempted with evil, and He himself tempts no one. But each person is tempted when

he [or she] is lured and enticed by his [or her] own desires." --James 1:13-14

God's plan of salvation was that Jesus was required to be beaten and killed so that we could be forgiven. This required His Son to die in our place, to take our punishment. Jesus volunteered to fulfill God's plan. Was Satan involved? Yes! John 13:2 said that during the last supper, the devil had already put it into the heart of Judas Iscariot to betray Jesus. God used Satan as His agent to complete this plan of salvation. Jesus suffered during the execution of God's plan. The disciples also suffered upon completion of the plan. But this suffering produced great benefits for mankind. God's plan will be fulfilled.

Since the fall, all people have a tendency towards evil. We must understand that God never commits evil. God uses the evil that Satan doles out and works it out for the good of those who love Him. He does this by interweaving that evil into His plan and purpose for good. The pain resulting from that evil has a purpose. Some pastors deny that God allows evil; they say God is love – and He is. However, if we say that God does not use Satan as His agent to fulfill His plans and purposes, then we have to admit that God is not all-powerful and in control. That means that Satan is more powerful, or at last equal to God, meaning God is powerless to deal with evil.

We are blessed to have a God that is all-powerful and in control. In the Garden of Eden, Satan was successful in getting God's perfect creation to sin. The sin caused all born on earth to have a sin nature that separates us from God and glorifies Satan.

God's divine plan is to allow all people to be forgiven and reconciled to God – if they choose to accept it.

God instituted a way to be forgiven with the Law and the sacrificial system. He did this to show the people that they were sinners and that they were in need of forgiveness. But the forgiveness was only temporary. A sacrifice was required every year. Paul, in his letter to the Romans, tells them, that the consequence of sin is death, spiritual and eventual physical death – separation from God. The writer of Hebrews tells us that without the shedding of blood, there is no forgiveness. In the Old Testament, God required a sinner to sacrifice an unblemished animal to die in their place. The animal was required to be perfect with no blemishes. God wanted to have the sinner lose something of value for a deeper impact. The animal was to be killed as a substitution for the sinner. The animal died for their sin. Imagine how many animals were killed for people's bad behavior. This was the forerunner to the New Covenant that Jesus initiated. God wanted to have a sacrifice that would be permanent forgiveness.

The New Covenant required a sinless - perfect person to be sacrificed for the sins of every person on earth. The problem – there are no perfect human beings. God's problem was that without the shedding of blood from a perfect unblemished human being, there could be no sacrifice – no forgiveness. A sacrifice was required. God is a spirit; a spirit cannot die. He needed a human being to complete His plan to forgive all people on Earth. God's plan was to send his Son to earth to be born of a human; the result – a God/man. Through the virgin birth, Jesus was fully human being, and fully God in one.

During Jesus' life, He experienced all the worst this world has to offer, all the same things we go through every day. He knows how difficult it is to live in a world under Satan's rule. He endured hunger, grief, physical pain, depression, and betrayal. He was betrayed by Judas, one of His followers. I'm sure Satan believed that he was going to kill the Son of God and he would win the war. Judas made his own choice to betray Jesus. God allowed Satan to enter Judas (Luke 22:3). We later find out that Judas was not a true follower. He had an evil heart and even stole money meant for the poor. He expected Jesus to rise up and battle the Romans and be a worldly king, he was wrong. Satan played on this and Judas' greed.

The Pharisees were the Jewish religious elite, they held powerful positions in the community. They were revered and received preferential treatment in the community. They were afraid of Jesus because they saw that He was admired and had the favor of God. They most likely knew that Jesus was who He claimed to be, but they also knew that Jesus would expose them as hypocrites. If exposed, they would then lose their positions of power. It was this arrogance and pride that fueled their thoughts of killing Jesus. Jesus was a good man; He did nothing to deserve death. Through false charges and pressure from the Pharisees, the Romans crucified Jesus. The Romans did not believe in the God of Israel, they just wanted to oppress the Jews. If Jesus died, the Pharisees would retain their powerful positions of respect and authority. Satan would chalk this up for a win against God.

God could have stopped the murder of His Son at any time. But He knew that without Jesus' death and resurrection, His plan of redemption could not be carried out.

In orchestrating this plan, God used the power-hungry Pharisees and the Romans to fulfill His plan of Jesus' suffering and death. Every painful event that Jesus endured was part of the divine plan. Isaiah 53:4-7 says,

> "Surely, He [Jesus] has borne our griefs and carried our sorrows; yet we esteemed Him stricken, smitten by God, and afflicted. But He was pierced for our transgressions; He was crushed for our iniquities; upon Him was the chastisement that brought us peace, and with His wounds, we are healed. All we like sheep have gone astray; we have turned—everyone—to his own way; and the LORD has laid on Him the iniquity of us all. He was oppressed, and He was afflicted, yet He opened not His mouth; like a lamb that is led to the slaughter, and like a sheep that before its shearers is silent, so He opened not his mouth."

After Jesus was beaten within an inch of His life, He was hung on the cross. This was a brutal way to kill someone. The nails through His hands and feet were not the most painful experience He endured; it was the sins of the world. As Jesus hung on the cross, God imputed onto Him all the sins of all the people of the earth. Your sins, my sins, our ancestor's sins, past, present, and future. As He took our sins upon Him, He experienced every pain that humans have ever felt. He was now a sinner, although He never sinned – it was our sins – not His.

He substituted Himself for us. That beating and death were meant for you and me. But because of His great love for us – He took it all for us. As God placed all our sins onto Jesus, God had to turn away from His Son. God hates sin, even the sin placed onto Jesus. Jesus felt abandoned, before His death, Jesus cried with a loud voice, "My God, My God, why have you forsaken me?" This is the worst pain of all- being separated from God. When He died, His mission was completed.

Every human being has been forgiven for all their sins – past, present, and future. All we need to do is accept the forgiveness. God fulfilled His divine plan for salvation, even at the pain and suffering of His Son. If Jesus' sacrifice had not occurred, there would be no permanent forgiveness, we would still be sacrificing animals in our backyards. The fulfillment of this plan brought peace and contentment into the world.

There is no use to fight Him, God's plan and purpose will be done – with or without you. Proverbs 16:9 says, "The heart of man plans his way, but the LORD establishes his steps," and 19:21 says, "Many are the plans in the mind of a man, but it is the purpose of the LORD that will stand." And lastly, Proverbs 16:4 says, "The LORD has made everything for its purpose, even the wicked for the day of trouble." God has a plan for believers and non-believers, you can be a part of that plan willing, or you can fight every step of the way. One way or another, God's plan will prevail. Your participation determines how much pain you will be required to endure. When you submit to God's plan, you have the promise that God will be there with you, helping you through your pain. When you are through the trial, I guarantee that you come out of it better than before – God works everything for the good!

2. GOD'S DISCIPLINE

> "Some were fools through their sinful ways, and because of their iniquities suffered affliction…" --Psalm 107:17

It is only through painful trials that we change our behavior. God's intention is to not only change your behavior but your character also. God changes your heart. By changing your heart – your behavior changes. Your beliefs dictate your behavior. God, through his Holy Spirit, changes your beliefs by transforming your mind into being aligned with the mind of Christ. This changes your character and behavior to conform to God's will.

Sin is anything that goes against God's moral standards. What are His moral standards? Jesus said it best in Matthew 22:36-40, the Jewish religious elite asked Jesus,

> "What is the greatest commandment?" Jesus replied, "You shall love the LORD God with all your heart and with all your soul and with all your mind. This is the great and first commandment. And the second is like it: you shall love your neighbor as yourself."

These are the only rules that Christians are commanded to follow – love God and everyone else. If you love someone, you cannot lie to them, steal from them, cheat on them, or judge them. If you love others, you will forgive them, humble yourself, you will be patient and kind to everyone, and place their needs above your own. Sinful behavior is not of love – it's selfish and prideful.

It is not like we don't know right from wrong - it's written in our hearts. James 4:17 says that if you know the right thing to do but do not do it, it is a sin. Sin results in consequences – discipline. Paul said, "There will be tribulation and distress for every human being who does evil…" (Romans 2:9).

The writer of the Book of Hebrews talks about God's discipline,

> "And have you forgotten the exhortation that addresses you as sons? 'My son, do not regard lightly the discipline of the Lord, nor be weary when reproved by him. For the Lord disciplines the one he loves and chastises every son whom he receives.' It is for discipline that you have to endure. God is treating you as sons. For what son is there whom his father does not discipline? If you are left without discipline, in which all have participated, then you are illegitimate children and not sons. Besides this, we have had earthly fathers who disciplined us, and we respected them. Shall we not much more be subject to the Father of spirits and live? For they disciplined us for a short time as it seemed best to them, but he disciplines us for our good, that we may share his holiness. For the moment all discipline seems painful rather than pleasant, but later it yields the peaceful fruit of righteousness to those who have been trained by it." –Hebrews 12:5-11

God disciplines the ones He loves. This is not a sign of rejection – but of love. If you have made Jesus Christ your Lord and

Savior, God has adopted you into His family (Galatians 3: 23-29). If you are a parent, you love your children unconditionally. Let's say your teenage daughter goes with her friends to the mall. At the mall, she steals some clothes and gets arrested by security. The police book her into the Juvenile Hall.

As a parent, you are angry and disappointed in your child. But you don't stop loving them, or love them less. Your relationship is obviously strained. Their sin has caused a separation in your relationship. But she is your daughter; you will never love her less. Your relationship will remain on the rocks until she makes restitution. Restitution can be defined as making good for some injury. Making good requires her to confess what she had done (acknowledge her mistakes), repent her mistake (turn away from that behavior), and make restitution to the injured party (in this example: make things right financially or restitution could be just apologizing for your actions). Your daughter confesses, seeks forgiveness, repents, and pays the damages. After restitution has been completed, your relationship with your teenager is restored. There still may be consequences from the court.

This is the same with our relationship with God. He is our heavenly Father; He loves us more than we could ever understand. He loves our children more than we could. When we sin, we must confess that sin, repent of it, and make it right. Just as our parents disciplined us, our Heavenly Father must discipline our poor behavior. Often, discipline is painful.

I remember my dad's discipline; it was not fun, matter-a-fact, it was painful. But the pain only lasted a short time, it did make me a better person and taught me many life lessons that helped me raise my girls. Therefore, I am grateful for my dad's discipline. If you're reading this and thinking, "I've never had a difficult trial in my life." It may be that you have never been disciplined by our heavenly Father. You are either perfect, or, you may not be adopted into God's family. You have to re-evaluate your relationship with God. Have you made Jesus Christ your Lord and Savior? Do you walk in the Holy Spirit? Search your heart now – be honest. Now is the time to dedicate or rededicate your relationship with God. Confess and repent and draw closer to Him.

God hates sin. He cannot allow it by looking the other way. He hates sin because He knows that if left unrepented, it destroys lives. Habitual sin causes pain, isolation, fear, shame, and emotional turmoil. Unrepented sin is the cause of emotional pain and suffering. Sin opens the door to Satan's oppression. God loves us too much to ignore our sins. He wants you to share in His holiness. Merriam-Webster defines "holy" as having a divine quality or being separated out of the world for God. He chooses you out of those who are not holy. Becoming holy is called the process of "sanctification." Sanctification is the ongoing process of aligning with God's will. This lesson is taught throughout the bible,

> "Before I was afflicted, I went astray, but now I keep Your word." --Psalm 119:67

> "It is good for me that I was afflicted, that I might learn Your statutes." --Psalm 119:77

God tells us we must endure discipline. It is the way we respond to discipline that causes pain, "My people are destroyed for lack of knowledge…" (Hosea 4:6). God knows that we are not faithful, we don't love God as we should, we lie, cheat, steal, and hate. This is because we don't know or understand who God is – we have no knowledge of God.

The Book of Hosea tells of God's enduring love for Israel, even though they consistently serve other gods. The Bible depicts God's people as His bride. A consistent theme throughout the bible tells how God's bride commits adultery by seeking out other gods and serving them. The Israelites enter into a cycle of sin, return to God, then sin again, each time suffering discipline. In chapter five, Israel had forsaken God once again. God pronounces His verdict on Israel. God said Israel's sins had separated them from Himself. Due to their sin, He allowed the Israelites to be taken into slavery by the Assyrians. He will place them into slavery until they acknowledge their sin and turn back to Him. It is only in our distress that we earnestly seek God. Hosea10:10 says,

> "When I [God] please, I will discipline them [Israel], and nations shall be gathered against them when they are bound up for their double iniquity."

Hosea 10:13 adds,

> "You [Israel] have plowed iniquity [sin]; you have reaped injustice; you have eaten the fruit of lies. Because you have trusted in your own way…"

In chapter fourteen, we see that Israel repents, and God restores them. Our confession and repentance reconciles our relationship. God loves us and always forgives our sins when we humble ourselves and seek Him. Restoration and healing occur at repentance. The book ends with,

> "Whoever is wise, let him understand these things; whoever is discerning let them know them; for the ways of the LORD are right, and the upright walk in them, but transgressors [sinners] stumble in them." --Hosea 14:9.

God can use a wide variety of people or situations to bring disciple. In Hosea, God used the pharaoh and the king of Assyria to discipline the Israelites. He could just as well use your neighbor, Satan, or your employer as His agents to enact discipline.

The Bible provides many examples of people suffering because of their sins. But we learn that God does not keep us in pain any longer than necessary to bring us to repentance. In the Old Testament, God told King Solomon,

> "If my people who are called by my name humble themselves, and pray and seek my face and turn from their wicked ways, then I will hear from heaven and will forgive their sin and heal their land." --2 Chronicles 7:14.

Humbling one's self, confession, and repentance is the key to shortening your discipline and restoring your relationship with God.

In the New Testament, we see a correlation between sin and illness. The Apostle John tells a story in John chapter five where Jesus and His disciples were in Jerusalem for a Jewish feast. As they walked past the pool of Bethesda, they saw a man who had been an invalid for twenty years. It was a tradition that when the water in the pool was stirred up, it was believed that angels were stirring up the water. It was thought that the first person to enter the water would be healed of all disease. There were many sick and diseased people who waited by the pool for the water to show some movement. Jesus asked the man if he wanted to be healed. The man responded that he was an invalid and could not get to the water fast enough when it was stirred. Jesus healed the man. The man then got up and walked off. Jesus later saw the man in the Temple and said, "See, you are well! Sin no more, that nothing worse may happen to you." This comment by Jesus suggests that one of the consequences of sin is illness.

It is very important to understand that sin has consequences, sin gives authority to Satan to oppress us. Satan's intent is to harm you. Satan's influence can include encouraging you to make poor decisions that will place you into sin, influencing unforgiveness, or being judgmental. God is in control. Satan cannot inflict pain or disease without God's permission. Repentance closes the door to Satan's oppression and restores that hedge of protection that He gives His children. Whether God allows Satan to inflict you with a trial in your life, or God brings it Himself, trust God's word in Romans 8:28, "…for those who love God all things work together for good…"

The Bible teaches that God allows and sometimes brings painful events into your life as discipline for sinful behavior. God disciplines the ones He loves. His love is a perfecting kind of love, not a pampering type of love that we get from grandparents. Discipline is for both training and teaching. Those of us who are parents do the same with our children. Discipline is for long-term benefit. God's discipline is not punishment, although sometimes it feels like it. Punishment is punitive. Discipline is training and teaching. Jesus took the punishment that was meant for you and me on the cross two thousand years ago.

3. FOR GOD'S GLORY

"… whether you eat or drink, or whatever you do, do all to the glory of God." --1 Corinthians 10:31

The primary purpose of human beings is to glorify God. This is done through praise, worship, and prayer, but primarily by our walk – the example we set for others, and by our testimony of how God has blessed us. People watch and evaluate others – especially Christians; what we say, what we do, how we treat others, and how we handle adversity. There are a lot of people who watch Christians in a-plan effort to call them out for their worldly behavior. They enjoy revealing hypocrisy – especially in the Christian community. Jesus taught,

"You are the light of the world. A city set on a hill cannot be hidden. Nor do people light a lamp and put it under a basket, but on a stand, and it gives light to all in the house. In the same way, let your light shine before others, so that they may see your good works and give glory to your Father who is in heaven." --Matthew 5:14-16

Christians are a light in the darkness. In the Bible, darkness refers to evil; the light represents good. Jesus added that if non-believers see the love that Christians exhibit, they will know that the love of God is in them. Our love, ethical behavior, and positive attitude is a light that shines bright in this evil world. It is this light that draws non-believers to the light of Jesus. It is our example that draws others to Christianity.

It is also through our testimony of God's mercy, grace, and love that brings others to God. King David said,

> "Oh sing to the LORD a new song; sing to the LORD, all the earth! Sing to the LORD, bless his name; tell of his salvation from day to day. Declare his glory among the nations, His marvelous works among all the peoples! For great is the LORD, and greatly to be praised; he is to be feared above all gods." --Psalm 96:1-3

When you declare His glory, you sow the seed in a non-believer's heart. When they see the love God has shown you, they will also want what you have. God will produce the growth in that seed. Testimonies build faith in other Christians; we all need a fresh injection of faith. Your testimony builds faith in others.

The Babylonian king Nebuchadnezzar attacked and conquered Jerusalem. The king exiled many Jews and took many captives to Babylon. A young prophet named Daniel was one of those exiled to Babylon. Daniel was devout and God blessed him by promoting him to be a governmental assistant. After King Nebuchadnezzar's death, King Darius began his reign. Darius made Daniel one of three regional presidents within the kingdom. This was a trusted position. Daniel was well respected by Darius and was being groomed to be the king's second in command. The scriptures say that Daniel had "an excellent spirit in him." God was working in Daniel's life.

The other governmental officers and assistants were jealous of Daniel. They resented that an exiled Jew had so much power. These men conspired to bring Daniel down – to have him killed. They watched and searched for faults but could not find any fault or corruption in Daniel. They saw that Daniel prayed to his God several times a day in public. The Babylonians did not believe in the God of Israel. They all decided that if they wanted to get rid of Daniel, they would have to use religion against him.

These conspirators got together and agreed to establish a new law that would target Daniel. The new law would prohibit praying to anyone or thing other than King Darius for thirty days. The punishment for violating this law would be death by the lion's den. The men tricked Darius into signing this new law by playing on the king's vanity.

Being fed to the lions was one of the worst forms of execution. The lions were starved prior to the execution to make them hungry and mean. Anyone who entered the lion's den would be attacked and eaten by the lions.

When Daniel found out about this law, he went to his house to pray. He went to his upper room and opened the windows for all to see. He faced Jerusalem, got on his knees, and prayed as he had done his entire life. The corrupt officials were watching him and saw him praying. Daniel could have conformed to the new law or even prayed in secret, but that would have been placing the king's will above God's will. Daniels's response to this new law was to pray more.

Daniel's enemies went to the king to report what they saw. They accused Daniel and suggested that he could not be trusted with the king's business. When the king heard his news, he was distressed and angry. The text does not explain why, but it may have been that he respected Daniel and was disappointed in Daniel for not following his law. Or, maybe he realized that he had been manipulated. The king was forced to punish Daniel, but his conscience bothered him that day.

Daniel's accusers reminded the king that the law could not be changed. The king hesitated, but the death penalty must be carried out. The king ordered the execution by the lion's den. Historians believe that this "den" was a large underground cave carved into the ground. The lions were fed through a hole in the ceiling or possibly through a side door. Daniel was brought to the cave; the king told him, "Maybe your God, whom you serve continually, deliver you!" Daniel was thrown into the cave, and it was sealed closed.

The king returned to his palace for the night. His conscience bothered him so much that he could not eat or sleep. At sunrise, the king returned to the lion's den to check on Daniel. He cried out in anguish to Daniel asking if he survived the night. Daniel responded by praising the king and telling him that God sent an angel to shut the mouths of the lions because God found no fault in him. Daniel was not harmed, and the king was happy that Daniel was safe. Daniel made it through his trial because he trusted God.

The king ordered that all the conspirators, their wives, and children were to be thrown into the lion's den, and all were killed by the lions. They reaped what they sowed for their malicious accusations against an innocent man. Daniel's faithfulness was rewarded by victory over his enemies. King Darius put out a decree to all nations within the kingdom and all the earth,

> "I make a decree, that in all my royal dominion people are to tremble and fear before the God of Daniel, for He is the living God, enduring forever; His kingdom shall never be destroyed, and His dominion shall be to the end. He delivers and rescues; He works signs and wonders in heaven and on earth, He who has saved Daniel from the power of the lions." --Daniel 6:26-27

It was through Daniel's persecution of his religion and faith in God that placed him in a horrible trial facing imminent death that God demonstrated His love by delivering Daniel from harm to glorify God. It was through Daniel's trial that King Darius and, most likely, thousands of other people that they came to know the true living God. The king then gave his testimony of God's love to all nations and people on earth. It's true Daniel suffered during this trial; however, his suffering cannot be compared to the glory of thousands of new believers. One man's pain resulted in many people being saved. Daniel's reward is waiting for him in heaven.

In John chapter eleven, the Apostle John tells the story of when Jesus raised Lazarus from the dead. In a small village called Bethany, Jesus' friends Lazarus, Martha, and Mary lived. Lazarus contracted an illness. Martha sent word to Jesus that Lazarus was sick and, on his deathbed, with the intention that Jesus would come and heal Lazarus. Jesus and His disciples were across the Jordan River teaching, preaching, and healing. Bethany was about one full day's journey from where Jesus was staying. When Jesus heard about Lazarus' illness, He said, "This illness does not lead to death. It is for the glory of God, so that the Son of God may be glorified through it."

Jesus loved Lazarus, Mary, and Martha, but He decided to stay where He was for two more days. After two days, Jesus said, "Our friend Lazarus has fallen asleep, but I go to wake him." The disciples did not understand the comment about being asleep. Jesus said, "Lazarus has died, and for your sake, I am glad that I was not there, so that you may believe."

When Jesus arrived in Bethany, He was told that Lazarus had died and had been in a tomb for a few days (like He didn't already know – He is God!). Many Jews came from Jerusalem to mourn Lazarus and console the sisters. Martha met Jesus and said, "Lord, if You had been here, my brother would not have died. But even now I know that whatever You ask from God, God will give You." Jesus told Martha, "I am the resurrection and the life. Whoever believes in Me, though he die, yet shall he live, and everyone who lives and believes in Me shall never die. Do you believe this?" She answered yes. Mary came out to Jesus and fell at His feet weeping. Jesus saw that she was upset; the scripture says He was deeply moved and greatly troubled. Jesus wept with the people.

Jesus went to the tomb with the sisters, with all the mourners following. At the tomb, Jesus was moved with grief. Jesus told the men to roll the stone away from the opening of the tomb. Martha warned Jesus that her brother had been dead for a few days and that the body would stink. Jesus said, "Did I not tell you that if you believed, you would see the glory of God?" The mourners rolled the stone away, opening up the tomb. Jesus looked up towards heaven and said,

> "Father, I thank You that You have heard Me. I know that You always hear Me, *but I said this on account of the people standing around, that they may believe that You sent Me.*" --John 11:42 Emphasis mine

Then Jesus yelled out, "Lazarus come out!" Lazarus walked out of the tomb, still wrapped in the burial linen as was the custom during those days. Many believed in Jesus that day and were born again. Everything Jesus did that day glorified the Father. Jesus knew Lazarus was going to die, yet He remained where He preached until Lazarus was dead and buried so that no one could dispute the resurrection. He knew that the Father would be glorified by Lazarus' resurrection. Was Lazarus' death a result of God's will? I don't know, but I believe that Satan caused illness and eventual death, and God glorified Himself through that event. God did this by showing His power. Jesus prayed out loud so that all would hear. He didn't pray, "Please raise Lazarus from the dead." He just thanked the Father. Jesus has the authority and the ability to raise the dead without the Father. He simply told Lazarus to come out. Lazarus may have been in pain those last days, and his family suffered with their grief over his death. But all pain has a purpose. The purpose here was to glorify God, increase the family's faith, and bring new believers into God's kingdom. I can imagine that all the people at the cave that day traveled all over the world, spreading the good news of Jesus. I'm sure that their testimony brought many more to believe.

The last story I would like to use as an example is in John chapter nine. Jesus and His disciples had just left the temple. They walked past a beggar that had been blind since birth. The disciples asked Jesus, "Rabbi, who sinned, this man or his parents, that he was born blind?" Most people at that time believed that illness and death were either a result of generational sin or the individual's sin; and that God was punishing them for that sin. Jesus replied, "It was not this man who sinned or his parents, but that the works of God might be displayed in him." Jesus was telling His disciples that God allowed that man to be born blind so that when the time was right, Jesus would walk past and heal him so that God's power could be glorified.

It seems so unfair; this man suffered so much being blind at a time when handicapped people were shunned because the people believed they were unclean due to sin. This man lived in darkness until Jesus came by and healed him and showed him the light. After his healing, this man spread the news of his healing. So much so that the Jewish religious elite heard about it and questioned the beggar. His testimony led to countless people being saved.

In this world, you may never learn the purpose of your trial and suffering. I believe that when we finally go home to heaven, we will be told the reasons and shown the impact of our short time of suffering, and all things will fall into place. Until that time, you can be comforted that God loves you and will not allow you to experience any more pain than necessary to bring about God's plan and purpose. This promise of God is that all things will work for your good.

Whether or not your trial is for God's glory or another reason, you must still praise and worship God through this difficult time and thank Him for what He is doing in your life. Praise and worship will give you the strength to make it through your trial. Remember, what you believe is how you behave. If you believe that you are a child of God and that your pain has a purpose, you have hope. With hope, you will be able to stand tall and walk in God's promises. As others watch how you handle difficult times, their opinion of God is shaped. When a Christian goes through a painful trial trusting God, the result is a positive attitude. Non-believers are always watching Christians. They want to see how we behave during difficult times; a positive attitude gives others inspiration and hope. A negative attitude gives non-believers another reason to not believe in a living God. It is our testimony that provides the light in the darkness. If your trial has the purpose of glorifying God, rest assured that you will come out of that trial better than before.

4. GIVE YOUR TESTIMONY & INCREASE YOUR FAITH

Daniel 4-2

Your testimony is a very powerful tool. Testimony is defined as a statement given as evidence. Your testimony is simply a story – your story of what God has done in your life. Trials in your life give testimonies of God's power and goodness. Without a painful event, there would be no testimony. When you tell others of the wonderful way God brought you through an overwhelming life event, you provide them evidence that we have a loving God, believers increase their faith, and non-believers have a seed planted.

Your testimony will minister to someone who is in need, maybe even someone who is going through a similar trial. Paul tells us in Second Corinthians 1:3-4,

> "Blessed be the God and Father of our Lord Jesus Christ, the Father of mercies and God of all comfort, who comforts us in all our affliction, so that we may be able to comfort those who are in any affliction, with the comfort with which we ourselves are comforted by God."

This is all part of God's plan, to train Christians to help anyone who is in need. Remember, we are God's hands and feet here on earth to do His will. Without that trial in your life, you cannot know how to comfort others. We receive the most comfort from those who have been-there-and-done-that.

It is the will of God to give your testimony of comfort, deliverance, redemption, and salvation. King David shows this in Psalm 105:2 which says, "Sing to Him [God], sing praises to Him; tell of all His wondrous works!"

God will strategically place people in your path so you can tell others how God moved in your life -- take advantage of it. Begin by telling them about the difficult trial that came into your life and how painful it was. Describe how God intervened and gave you victory over the situation, how He healed your wounds, and what it taught you—no need to have a written script – no need for theological terms or doctrines. Just tell your story in your own words. What if God allowed your trial so that your victory would help just one person make it through their trial? Without your help, this person would be lost.

Do not underestimate the power of your story. Testimonies can change hearts; and through your story, glorify God. The Apostle Mark describes a time when Jesus delivered a man from demon possession. This man was possessed by many demons and lived in a graveyard far away from the other people. This man must have been acting crazy because the people tried to bind him in chains and shackles, but he was so strong that he broke them. This man lived in the graveyard and acted out by cutting himself with sharp rocks. Jesus ordered the demons out of the man. The text tells us that the man came into his right mind. The man was so happy that he wanted to follow Jesus as a disciple, he asked Jesus if he could follow Him. Jesus said, "Go home to your friends and tell them how much the Lord has done for you, and how He has had mercy on you" (Mark 5:1-20). Through your story, like his, God is glorified.

You may think that you are not good enough to talk to people about God. Your past is too messed up, too many poor decisions and mistakes; no one will listen to you. But God chose you to deliver His message to others through your testimony. First Corinthians 1:26-31 says,

> "For consider your calling, brothers: not many of you were wise according to worldly standards, not many were powerful, not many were of noble birth. But God chose what is foolish in the world to shame the wise; God chose what is weak in the world to shame the strong; God chose what is low and despised in the world, even things that are not, to bring to nothing things that are, so that no human being might boast in the presence of God. And because of Him, you are in Christ Jesus, who became to us wisdom from God, righteousness and sanctification and redemption, so that, as it is written, 'Let the one who boasts, boast in the Lord.'"

God often uses broken people: victims of abuse, abandoned, neglected, marginalized people, prison inmates, homeless, and other traumatized people to deliver His message to the world. Jesus chose His twelve disciples; they were not rich, or powerful, they were not kings, princes, priests, or even well-educated men; they were common hardworking men. Each disciple had their faults, but God uses people like them – like us to do His work. The world calls us broken, flawed, damaged goods, low-life's, but God calls us His children, His chosen saints! He chose you through His grace, not because of the things you have done, have not done, or how good you thought you were.

I met a man who gave me his wonderful testimony. He was an alcoholic; he told me that one day he was drinking because of all the bad things that he perceived happened in his life. As he sat drinking and watching television in his living room, the thought of suicide came into his mind. He went and got a loaded handgun from his bedroom. As he sat there building up his strength to kill himself, there was a pastor walking up his street. The pastor felt the Holy Spirit telling him to go to that house and tell the man inside that Jesus loves him. After a bit of debate with the Spirit of God, the pastor went to this man's door and knocked. The depressed man answered the door. The pastor told him that God asked him to tell the occupant that Jesus loves him. The man broke down crying. The two men went inside and spoke. The pastor told the man of Jesus' love. The drunk man accepted Jesus as his Lord and Savior. The man now helps alcoholics and speaks in churches about how God heals those in pain. Both men went out and told all who would listen about God's love.

Part of our testimony is the way we behave. For sixteen years of my career, I worked undercover. The objective was to blend into the environment. I dressed like a "biker" to blend into that world. I dressed as a construction worker to blend into that scene. And I even dressed in a suit to fit into that world. It was like living a double life. On one hand, I was me – a cop, but on the other, I was "Gary" – a drug dealer.

It's funny; many Christians are the same. They live a double life. Jesus' brother James describes this as being "double-minded." On Sunday, they go to church with the family carrying a Bible. But Monday through Saturday, they are undercover Christians. No one would guess that they were Christians by watching them or listening to their speech. They blend into the "world," which is led by Satan. Jesus spoke about these people in the Book of Revelation,

> "I [Jesus] know your works: you are neither cold nor hot. Would that you were either cold or hot! So, because you are lukewarm, and neither hot nor cold, I will spit you out of My mouth." --Revelation 3:15-16

Jesus said, "I know your works." He sees how you behave; He knows your heart. Some translations have vomit instead of spit. This is how Jesus feels about those who fake it and do not fully trust in Him and submit to Him. If we are grateful for all that God has done in our lives, how can we not follow Jesus and submit to Him.

It is important how we behave, if we do not act in a moral or ethical manner, we are no different than anyone else. We have no testimony. But when we make every effort to do the right thing, we send out a message, and people see Jesus in us, it glorifies God.

Testimonies increase faith. When you give your testimony, the hearer's faith in God is increased because they know a real person who has been blessed by God. The Apostle James explains this,

"Count it all joy, my brothers, when you meet trials of various kinds, for you know that the testing of your faith produces steadfastness. And let steadfastness have its full effect, that you may be perfect and complete, lacking in nothing." --James 1:2-4

God wants to prepare you for eternity. He wants you to be conformed to His Son, Jesus.

Stand proud! Do not be intimidated. Tell your story to those whom God put in your path. God put them in your path for a reason, to hear what you have to say. Tell everyone about the wonderful things that God has done for you, to you, and through you. When you share your testimony, you plant the seed of the gospel in their heart. In doing so, you are fulfilling another command of Jesus; Acts 1:8 says, "…you will be My witnesses in Jerusalem and in all Judea and Samaria and to the end of the earth." This is called the Great Commission. We are commissioned to spread God's word to all people; this is done through regular people who give their testimonies. BE BOLD! Share your testimony with someone today!

5. BRING YOU CLOSER TO GOD

"You [God] have made me see many troubles and calamities will revive me again; from the depths of the earth, you will bring me up again. You will increase my greatness and comfort me again." --Psalm 71:20-12

God allows trials in our lives to bring us closer to Him. A painful trial often drives us closer to our creator. Suffering often forces us to examine ourselves and refocuses our priorities and direction to see what is truly important in life. This often forces us to make adjustments and reset priorities, and hopefully, repent bringing us closer to God. We seek the comfort that only a loving God can provide. As we go through the pain and suffering of an overwhelming life event, we learn to lean on God and trust Him in the pain, and when He delivers, we draw closer to Him. When we do not seek God in our trials, we tend to respond to our pain in sinful ways, we become angry and bitter, depression sets in, we have a pity party, and we blame everyone but ourselves for our pain -- including God. It is our unrepented sin that keeps us in our pain, and the term of the trial is increased, and the pain is more intense.

As we draw closer to God, we recognize the blessings in our lives; we experience God's love. We can always trust in God's promises. Romans 8:28-29 says,

> "And we know that for those who love God all things work together for good, for those who are called according to His purpose. For those whom He foreknew, He also predestined to be conformed to the image of His Son…"

God promises us that even though we are in pain and things look like they will never be the same, even though we do not understand the reasons for our pain, and even though we feel that it is unfair, He will make our pain and suffering something that initiates growth and wisdom. God is doing great work in you, you may not see it now, but you will come out of your trial better than you ever would have imagined. After we have been through the trial, we look back at the trial and see we become better having experienced it. Trials mold us and shape us into the people we are today. Who gets better by experiencing good times?

Knowing and understanding this doesn't make the pain any easier. But we know that God is with us every step of the trial to comfort us, and to promote us after we have persevered. Psalm 23 comforts us,

> "The LORD is my shepherd; I shall not want. He makes me lie down in green pastures. He leads me by still waters. He restores my soul. He leads me in paths of righteousness for His namesake. Even though I walk through the valley of the shadow of death, I will fear no evil, for You are with me; Your rod and staff comfort me. You prepare a table before me in the presence of my enemies; You anoint my head with oil; my cup overflows. Surely goodness and mercy shall follow me all the days of my life, and I shall dwell in the house of the LORD forever."

I am a great example of God drawing me into a closer relationship with Him. I never believed in God, I always did things on my own and only trusted in myself. After experiencing many traumatic events in my job as a police officer, I was diagnosed with PTSD. I was then diagnosed with an incurable debilitating neuro-muscular disease that caused me great emotional pain; after thirty surgeries on my feet, I developed an opioid addiction; and finally, my daughter came down with a serious illness. I responded with sinful behavior. I made sinful inner vows, judgments, and expectancies that led me to isolate myself from friends and family and kept me in pain. This all led me to make bad decisions that led me to a prison sentence. After my arrest, God put people in my path to tell me the gospel. Thank God I responded. What Satan meant for evil, God turned into something good. After giving my life to Jesus Christ, God healed my daughter, He put me in positions to learn more about Him, He healed my PTSD, and He revealed His plan and purpose in my life. God blessed me in many ways – He changed my heart and showed me to look at life from His perspective. I now have the peace and joy that I have never experienced. I give my full testimony in my book, *"Christ Centered Healing of Trauma: Healing a Broken Heart."* In the book, I teach how to heal the trauma in your life.

God has a plan and purpose for your life; this plan was conceived before you were born (Psalm 139:13 & Ephesians 1:1-5). Satan wants to lead us astray – away from God by influencing us to ignore God's moral standards, which separate us from God. God's primary plan is to prepare each one of us for His coming kingdom. In order to complete this plan, God must draw you back to the family. God uses trauma and overwhelming life events to fulfill this plan. When we are in pain, we seek out our loving creator. When all is going well, and we are prosperous, we do not seek God. Those who endure and persevere through the trials will experience the greatest blessing possible – eternal life in heaven.

It's all about perspective. Those who do not believe in God will ask questions about suffering and believe that life is not fair. Christians who have been through or are now going through trials will see our pain through a different lens. We see purpose in our pain and see how God brought us back into the fold, as Jesus talks about the one sheep out of the 99 (Matthew 18:12-14). If we look at our pain from God's perspective - when we come out of the trial, we see God's fingerprints all over our pain. Compare this to non-believers who do not believe in a creator, if there is no God, no creator. No creator, no creation. No creation, no purpose. If our pain is merely random, there is no purpose to the pain. Thus, no hope for the future. But we have hope, that hope is in eternal life. When compared to eternal life in heaven, your pain today is insignificant. I'm not saying it is not real, but it is trivial compared to what is in store for us.

If you're going through a trial at this time and have not fully committed your life to Jesus, please do it now; pray this prayer,

Father,

I confess that I am a sinner. I repent of my sins. I want to make Jesus Christ my Lord and Savior. He died on the cross for me so that my sins could be forgiven and that I would be healed. I believe that He was resurrected and now sits at Your right hand.

Father, I love You, and I thank You for calling me, loving me, and forgiving me. Thank You for Your mercy, grace, and healing.

In Jesus' name, I pray, Amen

Now that you've placed your trust in Jesus, instead of praying to get out of your trial, pray asking Him to tell you what He wants to change in you or what He wants you to learn. But there is a warning – don't ask unless you are prepared to accept and embrace what He tells you. Trust God, and He will be with you every step of your trial.

6. HUMBLING AND TESTING / REFINING

"If my people who are called by my name humble themselves, and pray and seek my face and turn from their wicked ways, then I will hear from heaven and will forgive their sin and heal their land." --2 Chronicles 7:14

HUMBLING

The Bible teaches that God allows us to go through painful trials to humble us. The Bible tells the story of the Israelites who were enslaved in Egypt for 400 hundred years. The story teaches God's purpose of testing and humbling. As the Israelites fled Egypt, God led them on their journey to the promised land by a cloud by day and a pillar of fire by night. When they were blocked at the Red Sea and the Egyptian army closed in on them, God parted the sea so they could cross on dry ground. When the nation had crossed, and the Egyptians were closing in, God restored the sea, causing the Egyptian army to drown. God demonstrated many miracles for the Israelites, but they never truly trusted God. In the desert, God fed them every day, made water come out of a rock, and their clothing did not wear out. With every sign of trial, the people complained and even suggested that their slavery was better than their freedom. Even though they witnessed many miracles, they did not trust God to take care of them. The trip from Egypt to Canaan was less than a month, but because of the people's disobedience to God, He led them around the wilderness traveling in circles for forty years. Deuteronomy 8:2 says,

> "You shall remember the whole way that the LORD your God has led you [Israelites] these forty years in the wilderness, that He might humble you, testing you to know what was in your heart, whether you would keep His commandments or not."

The Israelites failed the test; they would not humble themselves and trust God. As a punishment, God allowed them to wander around the wilderness until that entire disobedient generation had died off. Then He brought them into Canaan.

The topic of humility is a theme throughout the bible, some scriptures include,

> "The LORD lifts up the humble; He casts the wicked to the ground." --Psalm 147:6

> "When pride comes, then comes disgrace, but with the humble is wisdom." --Proverbs 11:2

> "He [God] has shown strength with his arm; He has scattered the proud in the thoughts of their hearts; He has brought down the mighty from their thrones and exalted those of humble estate…" --Luke 1:51-52

> "Humble yourselves before the Lord, and he will exalt you." --James 4:10

"Humble yourselves, therefore, under the mighty hand of God so that at the proper time He may exalt you…" --1 Peter 5:6

Another example is the story of Esther.

King Ahasuerus was the king of the Persian Empire in around 483 B.C.... The king promoted a man named Haman the Agagite (a descendant of the Amalekites) and set him above all the other officials. The Amalekites were enemies of the Jews. And all the king's servants who were at the king's gate bowed down and paid homage to Haman, for the king had so commanded them. But there was a Jewish man named Mordecai who did not bow down to Haman. Mordecai said he would not bow down to anyone except for God. When Haman saw that Mordecai did not bow down or pay homage to him, He was filled with fury because of his pride. Haman loved the attention and the adoration of the people.

He wanted to punish Mordecai for his insolence. Haman developed a plan to not only punish Mordecai but sought to wipe out all the Jews throughout the entire kingdom. One day Haman said to King Ahasuerus,

> "There is a certain people scattered abroad and dispersed among the peoples in all the provinces of your kingdom. Their laws are different from those of every other people, and they do not keep the king's laws so that it is not to the king's profit to tolerate them. If it pleases the king, let it be decreed that they be destroyed…"

The king took his signet ring from his hand and gave it to Haman. The king said to Haman, "The money is given to you, the people also, to do with them as it seems good to you."

The king's scribes were summoned, and a new law was written according to all that Haman commanded. The new law was sent to all the officials of all the peoples, to every province in its own language. It was written in the name of King Ahasuerus and sealed with the king's signet ring that was given to Haman. The law instructed the people that on a certain day, to kill every Jew, young and old, women, and children, and to steal their possessions.

Mordecai heard the plan and was deeply distressed. His relative Esther was the queen. He spoke to Esther and asked her to intercede for the Jews. This intercession was dangerous, but she realized that this was God's plan for her. Esther ordered all the Jews to fast and pray for three days for her success.

Esther's plan was to hold a feast for the king and Haman the next day. Haman went out of the palace that day joyful and glad of heart. But when Haman left, he saw that Mordecai did not bow before him and became filled with rage. This is what pride does, it puffs us up and causes us to believe we are better than we really are. Haman went home to his wife and friends and bragged to them about the splendor of his riches, all the promotions with which the king had honored him, and how the king placed him above the officials of the king. Haman said, "Even Queen Esther let no one, but I come with the king to the feast she prepared. And tomorrow also I am invited by her together with the king." His wife and all his friends said to him,

"Let a gallows 75 feet high be made, and in the morning, tell the king to have Mordecai hanged on it. Then go joyfully with the king to the feast." Haman was pleased with this idea. Haman ordered those large gallows be built especially for Mordecai.

Esther cooked the feast; the king and Haman ate. After the feast, they were drinking wine; the king asked Esther, "What is your wish, Queen Esther? It shall be granted you. And what is your request? Even to the half of my kingdom, it shall be fulfilled." Esther answered,

> "If I have found favor in your sight, O king, and if it pleases the king, let my life be granted me for my wish, and my people for my request. For we have been sold, I and my people, to be destroyed, to be killed, and to be annihilated. If we had been sold merely as slaves, men, and women, I would have been silent, for our affliction is not to be compared with the loss to the king."

Then King Ahasuerus answered the Queen, "Who is he, and where is he, who has dared to do this?" Esther responded, "A foe and enemy! This wicked Haman!" Then Haman was terrified before the King. You can see how God was using each biblical character to humble Haman.

The King was angry at Haman and walked out of the room to cool off, but Haman stayed to beg for his life from Esther. The King returned from the garden as Haman was sitting on the couch with Esther. And the King said, "Will he even assault the queen in my presence, in my own house?" One of the King's servants told the King that Haman had gallows built for

Mordecai and is standing at Haman's house, seventy-five feet high." The King said, "Hang him on that." They hanged Haman on the gallows that he had prepared for Mordecai. The King later promoted Mordecai to Haman's position, and the genocide was averted. Haman was so prideful that he was murderous. God needed to humble this man, he refused to be humbled, and God had to protect His people. There is so much more to the story of Esther. Everyone should read the book of Esther.

God is not a respecter of men. Even the Apostle Paul was allowed to suffer while doing great work for God. Paul had some sort of illness. In Second Corinthians 12:7-10 Paul says,

> "So, to keep me [Paul] from becoming conceited because of the surpassing greatness of the revelations, a thorn was given me in the flesh, a messenger of Satan to harass me, to keep me from becoming conceited. Three times I pleaded with the Lord about this, that it should leave me. But He said to me, 'My grace is sufficient for you, for my power is made perfect in weakness.' Therefore, I will boast all the more gladly of my weaknesses, so that the power of Christ may rest upon me. For the sake of Christ, then, I am content with weaknesses, insults, hardships, persecutions, and calamities. For when I am weak, then I am strong."

Paul said that he was suffering from some sort of illness or harassment from Satan. The Greek word for the word "harass" is "kolaphizō," which means to punch or to strike with a fist.

Even though Paul was in some sort of pain, God refused to heal His main Apostle to prevent Paul from becoming prideful.

TESTING

The story of Job shows that God can use others, including Satan, to test us. The book of Job teaches that God sets limitations on Satan. In the first chapter, we learn that God speaks to Satan in heaven. God bragged on Job, calling him, "A blameless and upright man, who fears God and turns away from evil." God was proud of Job. Satan, living up to his name as the "accuser," told God that Job was only praising Him because He blessed Job. God allowed Satan to test Job with a limitation that Satan was not allowed to injure Job. Satan had Job's entire family killed and had thieves steal all his wealth. When Job heard the bad news, he tore his robe and shaved his head (these are signs of mourning), he fell on the ground, and worshipped God. Job said,

> "Naked I came from my mother's womb, and naked I shall return. The LORD gave, and the LORD has taken away; blessed be the name of the LORD." --Job 1:21

Job did not sin or accuse God of wrongdoing. God and Satan met again; now God had reason to brag. Satan again accused Job of kissing up to God because God blessed him and gave him a hedge of protection. God allowed Satan to test Job again, this time with the limitation that Satan could do what he wanted but could not kill Job. Satan inflicted a disease on Job; there were sores all over his body. Job's wife said, "Do you still hold fast to your integrity? Curse God and die." Job responded,

"Shall we receive good from God, and shall we not receive evil?" Job did not sin against God. Job mourned for a very long time. Some friends came because they heard what had happened. They accused Job of sinning, and because of his sin was being punished, Job maintained his innocence.

Job cried out to God, asking why he was going through this trial. In chapter 38, God asks Job who he thinks he is when he asks "why?" God said that Job asks questions without knowing what he is talking about. God asks Job where were you? God created the heavens and earth! Basically, God tells Job He is sovereign over everything and everyone, and He has a reason for everything He does. Job finally responds, "I know that You can do all things, and that no purpose of Yours can be thwarted." Job then repents for doubting God; God restores Job's wealth and then doubles it. God gave him ten more children. He already had ten children waiting for him in heaven.

The lesson in this book is that God is sovereign. We must trust Him; He created all things and knows what is best for us. We do not need to know why God allows us to suffer, we just need to understand that God is in control of all things, that He loves us unconditionally, and will never give us more than we can handle.

REFINING

A byproduct of the humbling process, is our being refined in our faith. *Refine* is defined as: to clean from impurities or unwanted material, to free from moral imperfection, to free from what is coarse, or vulgar. God knows everything; He knows your heart. Jeremiah 17:10 says, "I the LORD search the heart and test the mind, to give every man according to his ways, according to the fruit of his deeds." We all believe that we are good people, we don't see ourselves as sinners. But our heart is evil, "The heart is deceitful above all things, and desperately sick; who can understand it?" (Jeremiah 17:9). Sin destroys lives, it hardens and callouses our hearts, "But exhort one another every day, as long as it is called 'today,' that none of you may be hardened by the deceitfulness of sin" (Hebrews 3:13). A hard heart remains in sin, sin causes havoc in our lives and blocks our healing and peace.

God's goal is to prepare us for eternity in heaven; He must refine us, make us better – soften our hearts. God uses pain and suffering to refine His chosen saints. If you're reading this, you are chosen by God to do good works. The Apostle Peter explains this,

> "In this, you rejoice, though now for a little while, if necessary, you have been grieved by various trials, so that the tested genuineness of your faith - more precious than gold that perishes though it is tested by fire - may be found to result in praise and glory and honor at the revelation of Jesus Christ." --1 Peter 1:6-7

Peter says we must be tested by fire. These tests are called "trial-by-fire." All valuable precious metals must be refined to be purified. *Pure* is defined as a substance that contains nothing that does not properly belong and is free from moral fault or guilt. Gold that is mined contains other metals like iron, nickel, and copper. The mined gold with its impurities, is hard and corrosive. As the impurities are removed, the gold becomes softer and pliable.

A very high heat must be used to purify precious metal. Metal like gold is placed in a pot or container and placed on top of the fire, soon, the metal liquefies. Impurities rise to the top of the liquid. At the proper time, the refiner skims off the impurities, being careful not to remove any of the precious metals. This process is repeated several times, each time turning up the heat a bit more. More impurities are removed. The refiner may place a piece of charcoal into the liquid. The charcoal brings out the metal's sheen. Soon the refiner's reflection will appear in the liquid. This is what God does in our lives, putting us through the heat of a trial until His reflection is seen in us. God chose us to be molded into the likeness of His Son. Romans 8:28-29 says,

> "And we know that for those who love God all things work together for good, for those who are called according to His purpose. For those whom He foreknew, He also predestined to be conformed to the image of His Son..."

And Hebrews 2:10 adds,

"For it is fitting that He [Jesus], for whom and by whom all things exist, in the bringing many sons to glory, should make the founder of their salvation perfect through suffering."

If Jesus was made perfect through His suffering, we may expect the same suffering to refine and perfect us for the day we are glorified.

God is the refiner. When He sees impurities in us, He turns up the heat. Maybe He sees that we have too much pride, and He turns up the heat to humble us. If we become addicted to a sinful habit, He will turn up the heat, so we seek out His help. Maybe, He sees us running away from Him acting as our own god; He places a trial in our lives to draw us closer to Him. During good and prosperous times, we do not seek out the comfort of God because we believe our success is from our own work, not God's. God may allow more than one trial in our life in order to bring us closer to the image of Jesus. James, the brother of Jesus, gives us great advice while going through a trial. James, 1:2-4 says,

"Count it all joy, my brothers, when you meet trials of various kinds, for you know that the testing of your faith produces steadfastness. And let steadfastness have its full effect that you may be perfect and complete, lacking nothing."

As we get through a trial, God says, "Behold, I have refined you, but not as silver; I have tried you in the furnace of affliction." (Isaiah 48:10). As I stated before, the trials that we go through cause a change in our lives. God will make sure these trails work for your good in some way. It is only you that can prevent the good from materializing.

We recognize that through our trials, we are trained in godliness. The dictionary defines train as to teach so as to make fit, qualified, or proficient; to form by instruction, discipline, and to make prepared. God wants to instruct and prepare us for entering the Kingdom of God. Normally, when we are called by Him to be His children, we are not familiar with God's word. As we grow closer to God, we learn more about Him and His divine plan for the world.

> "For the grace of God has appeared, bringing salvation for all people, training us to renounce ungodliness and worldly passions, and to live self-controlled, upright, and godly lives in the present age, waiting for our blessed hope, the appearing of the glory of our great God and Savior Jesus Christ…" --2 Timothy 4:11-13

> "If you put these things before the brothers, you will be a good servant of Christ Jesus, being trained in the words of the faith and of the good doctrine that you have followed. Have nothing to do with irreverent, silly myths. Rather train yourself for godliness; for while bodily training is of some value, godliness is of value in every way, as it holds promise for the present life and also for the life to come." --1 Timothy 4:6-8

Difficult times force us to seek out help from our creator. It is only through faith in God that we have the hope and strength to persevere. Knowledge builds faith. How do we gain knowledge? By reading the bible, listening to pastors teach the word, and following the leading of the Holy Spirit. Why do we need to learn more?

> "All Scripture is breathed out by God and profitable for teaching, for reproof, for correction, and for training in righteousness…" --2 Timothy 3:16-17

The word of God is profitable teaching and training in righteousness. Most people live their lives without God. They may believe in Him but do not make Him their Lord and Savior. These are called lukewarm Christians (Revelation 3:16). Lukewarm Christians are prime targets for God's instruction. Gaining wisdom is good; we should never stop learning about who God is and who we are in Christ.

7. TO GIVE US APPRECIATION OF LIFE / DO NOT BE CONFORMED TO THIS WORLD

The Bible teaches us that we are merely temporary visitors on this earth. At Jesus' second coming, Christians will be taken to their eternal home – heaven. The reason God does not want us to feel at home here is because Satan has control of *the world*. The world is a societal system under the control of Satan. practicing Christians should feel out of place on earth. We hope for the eternal, non-believers live for the hour. Our goals are different; we seek out doing good, but the world teaches us to be selfish. That's why Paul wrote in his letter to the Romans, "Do not be conformed to this world but be transformed by the renewal of your mind, that by testing you may discern what is the will of God, what is good and acceptable and perfect" (v.

12:2). Why not be conformed to the world? Because Paul knows that the world entices *the flesh*,

> "For the desires of the flesh are against the Spirit, and the desires of the Spirit are against the flesh, for these are opposed to each other, to keep you from doing the things you want to do…" --Galatians 5:17

Peter added,

> "Beloved, I urge you as sojourners and exiles to abstain from the passions of the flesh, which wage war against your soul." --1 Peter 2:11

This battle between *the flesh* and *the Spirit* is epic. What is the flesh? Paul doesn't mean our flesh and blood bodies. The flesh is our inner man, which is trained in rebellion by the world and Satan and will battle against us until we experience God's final antidote to the flesh: a resurrection body. The Spirit is the Holy Spirit that is given to all born-again Christians. So, we have a battle against good and evil. This battle causes inner turmoil that oppresses us and keeps us in emotional pain.

If God would remove all pain and suffering from this world, this would become our home, and we would get comfortable in it. This would result in us not wanting to leave this place and go to our eternal home.

We all have so much to be thankful for. Many would argue this, but I feel it is a true statement. It is very easy to get comfortable with our blessings, including the people in our lives. We take them for granted -- including God. Suffering can help us appreciate our blessings more fully. An illness can help us appreciate our good health. The loss of a loved one will make us appreciate those people in our lives that we no longer are able to be with. There are so many people and circumstances that we all need to be thankful for. But human nature and our flesh ignore others and promote self. We say I don't need anyone; I can do it myself. But all good things come from God, and we cannot do anything on our own, our hope is in Jesus.

CHAPTER EIGHT

HOW DO OTHER RELIGIONS DEAL WITH THE ISSUE OF SUFFERING?

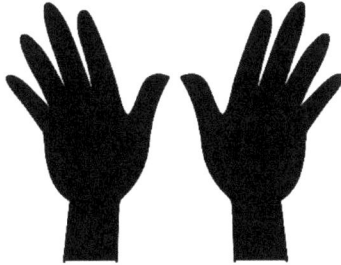

ISLAM

Let's take a look at how the three major religions handle the problem of suffering. We will begin with Islam. Islam teaches its followers to detach themselves from material possessions. It suggests that pain is brought on by attachments to things other than Allah (God). Islam states that when something good happens in your life, it is from Allah. If something bad happens in your life, it is a result of your actions. This is similar to the belief of the Old Testament people that if you do good, you will be blessed, do bad, and you will be cursed.

Islam teaches us to endure pain and suffering with hope and faith. The faithful are not counseled to resist it or to ask why. Instead, they accept it as God's will and live through it with faith that God never asks more of them than they can endure. Recognizing that their sin is the cause of their suffering, followers work to bring suffering to an end. The Islamic view is that righteous individuals are revealed not only through patient acceptance of their own suffering but through their good works for others. And if suffering is a consequence of sin, then good works will relieve pain.

The followers of Islam are taught to be indifferent to pain and suffering; they are to be grateful because it is good for the follower as pain removes sin. Followers believe that to be martyred in the name of Allah is considered noble, and they will be rewarded.

Islam has a series of rules to prevent sinning. These are called the Five Pillars:

1. Shahada is the declaration of faith and trust in Allah. Followers say this sentence in the Arabic language during prayer, "I bear witness there is no god to be worshiped but Allah and Muhammad are his servant and his messenger."

2. Salaat is prayer performed in Arabic language. Muslims may perform salaat anywhere at the time of prayer.

Salaat Consists Five Daily Prayers:

Fajr - means Dawn and beginning. Salaat is the first salat of the day and is performed at the dawn. Fajr prayer time starts from true dawn and ends at sunrise

Dhuhr - prayer is performed when sun declines

Asr - prayer is performed after dhuhr till when sun turns yellow

Maghrib - prayer time starts after the sun sets

Isha - may performed till midnight.

3. Sawm - the third Pillar of Islam Fasting. Allah prescribes daily fasting for all able and adult Muslims during the entire month of Ramadan (ninth month of lunar calendar). Followers must abstain from food, drink and sexual intercourse during the month of Ramadan, from dawn to sunset. This is mandatory for those who have reached puberty. Fasting helps develop self-control and grows patience. During the fast, a person learns to overcome their passions and desires in loving obedience to Allah. Fasting helps in strengthening one's faith.

4. Zakat - is a form of generosity that cleanses the soul. Zakat, by Quranic ranking, is next after prayer in importance. Zakat is binding on all believers who possess the means to do so. Zakat is based on savings, not income, and the value of all of one's possessions. These alms have restrictions and rules that must be abided.

5. Hajj - a journey to the annual Islamic pilgrimage to Makkah, the most holy city in the world. This is a mandatory religious duty for Muslims that must be carried out at least once in their lifetime by all adult Muslims who are physically and financially capable.

These pillars are meant to keep the follower's focus on Allah. Suffering only has meaning in regard to suffering for sin.

Source:

www.Islamicity.org

BUDDHISM

Buddhism is a religion that does not include the belief in a creator deity, or any eternal divine personal being. Buddhism has a different approach to that of Christianity, where the main goal of followers of the Buddhist faith is to escape the suffering that exists in the world. Buddha famously said that existence is suffering, and religion revolves around this premise. Buddhism teaches that the root cause of suffering is that humans lack the knowledge to relieve it, and the primary way to remedy is the Four Noble Truths, is the essence of Buddha's philosophies and outlines four stages of suffering.

The first Noble Truths Buddha diagnosed the problem of pain and suffering, and the second Noble Truth identifies its cause. The third Noble Truth is the realization that there is a cure, and the fourth Noble Truth is that there is an Eightfold Path to achieve a release from suffering.

Ultimately, the goal of Buddhism is to reach the end of all suffering. Buddhist believe this can be reached by following the teachings of the Four Noble Truths, and then the Eightfold Path, but also by living an ethical and spiritually aware lifestyle.

That is, everything is an effect of a cause. If the cause can be identified and destroyed, the effect is also destroyed." This mentality of diagnosing, understanding, and prescribing a cure to suffering, is what the Four Noble Truths focus on. The four Noble Truths are:

The First Noble Truth:

Suffering (Dukkha)

Suffering comes in many forms. Three obvious kinds of suffering correspond to the first three sights the Buddha saw on his first journey outside his palace: old age, sickness, and death. But according to the Buddha, the problem of suffering goes much deeper. Life is not ideal: it frequently fails to live up to our expectations. Fortunately, the Buddha's teachings do not end with suffering; rather, they go on to tell us what we can do about it and how to end it.

The Second Noble Truth:

Origin of suffering (Samudāya)

The Buddha taught that the root of all suffering is desire, tanhā. This comes in three forms, which he described as the Three Roots of Evil, or the Three Fires, or the Three Poisons.

These are the three ultimate causes of suffering:

1. Greed and desire, represented in art by a rooster

2. Ignorance or delusion, represented by a pig

3. Hatred and destructive urges, represented by a snake

The Third Noble Truth:

Cessation of suffering (Nirodha)

The Buddha taught that the way to extinguish desire, which causes suffering, is to liberate oneself from attachment. The Buddha was a living example that this is possible in a human lifetime.

The Fourth Noble Truth:

Path to the cessation of suffering (Magga)

The final Noble Truth is the Buddha's prescription for the end of suffering. This is a set of principles called the Eightfold Path. The Eightfold Path is also called the Middle Way: it avoids both indulgence and severe asceticism, neither of which the Buddha had found helpful in his search for enlightenment.

The eightfold path is at the heart of the middle road, which turns from extremes, and encourages us to seek a simple lifestyle. The eightfold path is Right Understanding, Right Intent, Right Speech, Right Action, Right Livelihood, Right Effort, Right Mindfulness, and Right Concentration. The meaning of "Right" has several aspects and includes an ethical and balanced middle road. When things go "right," we often experience a peaceful feeling inside, which confirms that we made the correct decision.

In Buddhism, the eightfold path is meant as a guideline to live life. Buddhism has nothing to do with faith; it seeks to promote learning and a process of self-discovery.

It is evident that Buddhism does not see suffering as a way to connect with God but as an opportunity to redeem one's self to escape the process of ongoing pain. This escape is done through detachment. The goal is to achieve a state where you do not desire anyone or anything. If you don't have an attachment to anything or anyone and do not desire anything or anyone, there can be no pain or suffering. Interestingly, this includes family and loved ones. If this is not achieved in your current life, you will be forced to repeat the same quest in your next life. This cycle will be repeated over and over until the State of Nirvana is obtained. In reality, Nirvana is a state that can never be achieved. Therefore, pain and suffering are your own fault, and there is no purpose to your pain except for punishment.

Source:

https://www.suffering-and-god.weebly.com/buddhism-views-on-suffering.html

https://www.bbc.co.uk/religion/religions/buddhism/beliefs/fournobletruths_1.html

HINDUISM

Hinduism is a polytheistic religion with an unknown and unnamed number of gods; many Hindus view the religion as a monotheistic religion with only one supreme being who is formless and impersonal. All other gods and goddesses are simply facets of this one god. This supreme being is viewed as the god of all other religions and equal to all existence or the ultimate reality. According to Hinduism, suffering is an inescapable and integral part of life. The goal of Hinduism is to resolve human suffering. As long as man is caught up in the worship of material possessions and becomes attached to them, there is no escape from suffering. Hinduism is a yearning for a lasting solution to the problem of human suffering. Hinduism focuses on the hidden causes of suffering and tries to resolve it by refining purity, balance, detachment, and indifference which liberates followers from suffering.

Hinduism identifies selfish behavior and selfish desires as the root cause of human suffering. When humans engage in selfish actions, they become vulnerable to suffering. Pleasure is not a solution to avoid pain. Desire comes from our attachment to anyone and anything. Hinduism promotes freedom from all kinds of desires and attachments by serving god and his creation, and is accomplished through various spiritual practices.

Hinduism acknowledges that while we may know the causes and possibly the solutions to suffering, suffering cannot be fully resolved as long as one is attached to worldly possessions and relationships. The purpose of Hinduism is not to end suffering, which is humanly impossible, but to learn to deal with it by reconditioning followers' minds and bodies. Followers must learn to endure suffering with detachment and acceptance, keeping faith in god and performing actions as an obligatory duty to god. Hinduism accepts karma as unavoidable; it acknowledges the importance of virtuous self-effort in shaping one's own destiny and correcting the wrongs of the past.

Hinduism teaches that karma should not make one hopeless, instead, it should make a person feel more responsible towards themself and their spiritual wellbeing, accepting suffering with an awareness that suffering is a result of their own behavior, and he/she has to be their own savior.

Source:

https://www.hinduwebsite.com/hinduism/h_suffering.asp

These religions address the problem of pain and suffering, however, do not answer the question. Christianity does answer the question and provides us with a Savior that provides forgiveness and cleanses us from our sins. In Christianity – your pain has a purpose.

CHAPTER NINE

PAIN

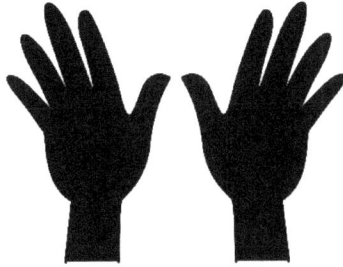

Christians should be comforted by the fact that there is always a purpose for pain and suffering. God often uses pain and suffering as a tool in our lives to mold, sharpen, and strengthen us - to mold you into the likeness of his son Jesus, to bring you closer to God and make you a better person, and to prepare you for the kingdom. Jesus talked about this, John 15:1-6 says,

> "I [Jesus] am the true vine, and My Father is the vinedresser. Every branch in Me that does not bear fruit [does good deeds] He takes away, and every branch that does bear fruit He prunes, that it may bear more fruit. Already you are clean because of the word that I have spoken to you. Abide in Me, and I in you. As the branch cannot bear fruit by itself unless it abides in the vine, neither can you, unless you abide in Me. I am the vine; you are the branches. Whoever abides in Me and I in him, he it is that bears much fruit, for apart from Me you can

do nothing. If anyone does not abide in Me, he is thrown away like a branch and withers; and the branches are gathered, thrown into the fire, and burned [hell]."

Jesus uses various metaphors to illustrate himself and his work. Water was not a safe drink in those days, most drank wine instead. Everyone was familiar with how to grow and maintain grapevines. Jesus is the genuine vine – the Messianic vine (Psalm 80:8). The Greek word for Branch, "klēma," comes from an old word from "klaō," meaning: offshoots of the vine, both words meaning tender and easily broken. The Word of God is a cleansing agent. It condemns sin, inspires you to strive for holiness, promotes growth, and it reveals God's power. The purpose of the branch is to bear fruit. People don't go through the trouble and work to raise grape vines to look at the pretty leaves; they want the sweet taste of the fruit. The analogy of fruit represents Christian character, such as the fruit of the Spirit in Galatians five. Service to God and society is possible only through abiding union with Jesus. Abide means: to accept without objection, to conform to, or to accept without objection. Abiding comes down to trusting Jesus and being obedient to Him.

Pruning grapevines is crucial if you want grapevines to be healthy and productive. Some vines can be left alone or only need light pruning. When left unpruned, grapevines become a tangled mess that looks unsightly and doesn't produce much fruit. Pruning is one of the most important things you can do for your plants. It's said that you can cut them back by 90%, and they'll be more productive than ever. Painful trials are often used to prune our poor character traits. Let us yield ourselves to be pruned by the Word of God, that we may not need the pruning of fiery trials.

"Those branches that do not bear fruit" means that either the cast-out branches are undercover (fake) Christians who never really abided in Jesus, and therefore go to hell; or that the fruitless Christians who live wasted lives also go to hell because of their fruitlessness. There is an easy way to avoid being one of the cast-out branches; have full trust, confidence, and assurance that Jesus is the Lord of your life. Real fruitfulness can only be determined over an extended period of time. Genuine conversion is not measured by belief in Jesus, even the evil spirits believe in Jesus, but they do not make Jesus their Lord and Savior. Fruitfulness is proven by long-term service to God.

We often define ourselves according to our pain; "I am an addict, a divorcee, a convicted felon, or I'm that guy with cancer." This is not your destiny. You are not your trauma, you are not your mistakes, or whom others say you are – you are a child of God. But Satan's lies try to convince you otherwise. Satan tells you that no one loves you – even God. Anger is toxic. This causes resentment and anger, that turns into a complaining spirit.

During my police career, I was truly scared in several situations where there was a person who intended to hurt me. There was no question of who my adversary was. But in the spiritual world, we cannot see our enemy; we can hear him. He says, "Your no good. Everyone knows your mistakes; they hate you." These are lies that Satan repeats to us every day.

I am grateful for police dispatchers who faithfully monitor the on-duty officers. I knew I could call for help at any time, and they would send help to me, however, I had to speak in terms they understood in regard to my needs. This is very similar to the prayers we cry out to God. God hears all your prayers, but we need to pray correctly. If we pray for God to remove our trial, we go against God's will. God either placed you in or allowed your trial. It is His will that you are where you are. Praying to remove God's plan and purpose will only prolong and deepen your pain -- it won't be answered. A better prayer would be asking God to provide you with wisdom and understanding for your pain and asking Him to teach you what He wants you to learn.

It is not uncommon to pray, asking God to remove your pain, Jesus did it. Matthew 26:39 records Jesus' prayer the night before His death, Jesus prayed, "My Father, if it be possible, let this cup pass from me; nevertheless, not as I will, but as you will." Jesus did not want to endure His trial because He knew it would require Him to suffer great amounts of pain. But Jesus knew God's plan and said, your will, not mine, be done. Through Jesus' suffering, we are no longer required to suffer for our sins.

Jesus purchased you with His blood; God will make something good out of our pain. Everything that happens is for His glory and your good. I believe there is a side to suffering we miss when we focus solely on our pain rather than on God's greater purpose. When you see the purpose behind the pain, you can find a way to endure it. If you can see the purpose beyond the pain, you will understand God's ability to leverage the suffering in your life for greater things. You cannot turn back time. You can't change the way you were raised; you cannot undo that bad decision, you can't change the economy, you can't change that person's opinion of you, but you can control your response and give these circumstances to God and trust there is a purpose to the pain.

The scripture does not state that you will simply suffer randomly, but that you suffer for the purpose of being molded into a better person, more importantly, that you persevere through that suffering. God does not orchestrate purposeless suffering in your life, but rather, redeems your suffering, giving you the wisdom to endure it for the purpose of serving as a witness to the power of the gospel. We need to always be aware that people, including our children, spouse, friends, enemies, and even skeptical nonbelievers - will observe the way we handle suffering, and they may come to repentance because of our example. When they see us endure the same kind of pain and overwhelming life events they experience while remaining humble, in faith, and prayerful before God, they will be curious about the source of our strength.

Scripture tells us, "We are afflicted in every way, but not crushed; perplexed, but not driven to despair; persecuted, but not forsaken; struck down, but not destroyed" (2 Corinthians 4:8-9). In these verses, Paul is referring to multiple types of suffering – mental, physical, emotional, and spiritual. When suffering comes, it can take a major toll on our spirit – breaks our hearts. It's important that we recognize that suffering is part of spiritual warfare.

For the Christian, suffering helps us to keep our eyes not on the temporal, but on things of eternal value, to have compassion on others, to prove to men the genuineness of our convictions, to develop patience, and to prove our love and loyalty towards God. It helps us to understand the heart of God better and to appreciate our blessings. First Peter 2:20-21 says, "But if you suffer for doing good and you endure it, this is commendable before God. To this, you were called, because Christ suffered for you, leaving you an example, that you should follow in his steps."

CHAPTER TEN
COMING OUT OF A TRIAL

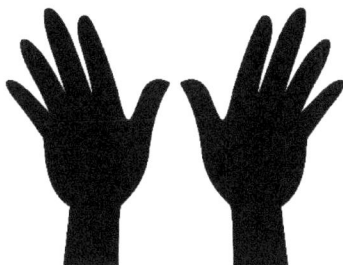

The question of 'Why does God allow suffering?' has been asked since creation. I have tried to answer this question as I understand it. However, can we truly know why God does what He does?

The lesson learned from the book of Job is that man does not and may never know the reason for the things that happen in his life. The book does not answer the problem of evil but does teach that it is impossible for finite man to fathom the secrets of an infinite God. Man can never understand the depths of God, and how God deals with each man. Man is encouraged to look steadfastly at the Lord, trust him, and be devoted to him because God is loving and merciful, and all of his purposes are part of his ultimate plan, which no one can understand.

But we continue to seek out answers to why God allows our pain. As with Job, do we really want to know the answer? Or do we only want to know that we are not alone in our pain? Job's friends tried to provide comfort, but as is human nature, we accuse others of being worse than we are. We cannot find comfort in the worldly experience. Our true comfort and peace comes only from a close relationship with God.

This is well illustrated in the story of Cain and Abel in Genesis 4:1-16. After Adam and Eve were banished from the garden, they had the first children born on Earth. The first son they named Cain, then his brother Abel was born. Cain was a farmer working crops, and Abel was a sheep herder. One day they both brought God an offering. Genesis 4:3-4, "Cain brought to the LORD an offering of the fruit of the ground, and Abel also brought of the firstborn of his flock and of their fat portions. And the LORD had regard for Abel and his offering, but for Cain and his offering he had no regard." God was pleased with Abel's offering but not with Cain's. It is not known why they gave this offering because God had not yet instituted the law, nor why God rejected Cain's offering.

Genesis continues, "So Cain was very angry, and his face fell. The LORD said to Cain, 'Why are you angry, and why has your face fallen? If you do well, will you not be accepted? And if you do not do well, sin is crouching at the door. Its desire is contrary to you, but you must rule over it'" (v. 5-7). Cain's facial expression showed what was in his heart. His anger was undoubtedly rooted in pride and envy. He couldn't bear that his brother was accepted before God, and he was not. It is even possible that this was public knowledge, envy, and shame are powerful motivators. Cain's anger is questioned by God. God is warning Cain that sin will destroy him – sin breeds more sin.

God is teaching Cain a valuable lesson. Sin is of the flesh and a result of Adam's sin. Sin wants to control us, but when in fellowship with God, we have the power to rule over it. The epidemic of sin is quickly becoming worse. Cain now commits the sin of spiritual pride and hypocrisy.

Soon after, Cain spoke to Abel in the field, Cain rose up against Abel and killed him. Sometime later, "…the LORD said to Cain, 'Where is Abel your brother?' He said, 'I do not know; am I my brother's keeper?' And the LORD said, 'What have you done? The voice of your brother's blood is crying to me from the ground. And now you are cursed from the ground, which has opened its mouth to receive your brother's blood from your hand. When you work the ground, it shall no longer yield to you its strength. You shall be a fugitive and a wanderer on the earth.' Cain said to the LORD, 'My punishment is greater than I can bear. Behold, you have driven me today away from the ground, and from your face, I shall be hidden. I shall be a fugitive and a wanderer on the earth, and whoever finds me will kill me.' Then the LORD said to him, 'Not so! If anyone kills Cain, vengeance shall be taken on him sevenfold.' And the LORD put a mark on Cain, lest any who found him should attack him."

The downward course of sin has progressed quickly, resulting in the murder of an innocent person. Cain said, "Am I my brother's keeper?" This reply of Cain is famous. The fact of the matter is that he was supposed to be his brother's keeper, but was instead his brother's murderer. He murdered him for no tangible reason; Able had not injured Cain in any way. Cain's murderous rage was inspired purely by jealousy. Sin has consequences, Cain's sin resulted in a curse. The curse was that similar to Adam, his work would be hard and would result in minimal results. Cain was banished from the place where he lived, as with Adam and Eve. He would now fear for his life daily. Other consequences include loss of fellowship and blessings from God and loss of protection and grace.

Cain didn't feel remorse about his sin, but only about his punishment. One of the clearest results of sin is our innate desire to justify our sin and complain if we are judged in any way. One of the consequences of sin is that it makes us pity ourselves instead of causing us to turn to God. One of the first signs of a saved person is that the individual takes sides with God against himself – humbling him or herself. Cain disappointed God by his sin, but God's love did not diminish. God marked Cain as His son – not to be harmed.

This story teaches that it is our response to negative events that dictate our future – growth or oppression. Cain was angry and envious of his brother; he may have even felt resentment towards God for his own behavior as his father.

Our behavior is based on what we believe. Cain believed he was given the short-end-of-stick. He was angry with Abel, that most likely turned into hatred. His belief led him to kill his brother. If he had said to himself, "I will bring a better offer next time." Or, possibly spoke to God asking why his offering was not well received, he could have prevented his bleak future and received blessings instead of a curse. The emotional pain you are experiencing is not from your trial; it is from your response to that trial. That response is the root cause of most emotional issues. Our default setting is to do all we can to stop the pain. This is normally attempted through any substance or activity that will dull and take your mind off the pain. We do not deal with the root issue because it is too painful. Our default coping mechanisms are usually sinful. Sin separates us from God and blocks our healing and blessings. It is our pride, self-centeredness, resentment, and bitterness that causes the pain. Your separation from God causes spiritual turmoil in our spirit. The only remedy is to restore your relationship with God. Our response to overwhelming painful events is extremely important and will result in blessings or curses.

You may have experienced a painful event in your past that still haunts you, or, you may be going through a painful trial right now; that pain is real, and it hurts – I know. It may not seem that there is a purpose to the pain, but God is in charge. Jesus knows what you're going through; He is with you right now. Jesus suffered through the same things we do. He grieved, He was hated, misunderstood, ridiculed, laughed at, and even His family thought He was crazy (Mark 3:20-21). There is nothing that you will go through that Jesus has not experienced. This is why you can be comforted that He will bring you through your trial(s) because He experienced the same pain.

Instead of focusing on what happened to you, or what someone did to you, consider the reason for your pain. What is God trying to accomplish? You may be part of a grand plan that requires you to suffer to achieve His plan and purpose. If so, are you a bit player, or do you have a lead role? Either way, you can be comforted that God loves you enough that He is using you to help Him with His plan. Submitting to God's will is finding peace – even in your pain, you can have peace and even joy. Believe me, I know it is not easy, it is often difficult, I know, I've been there.

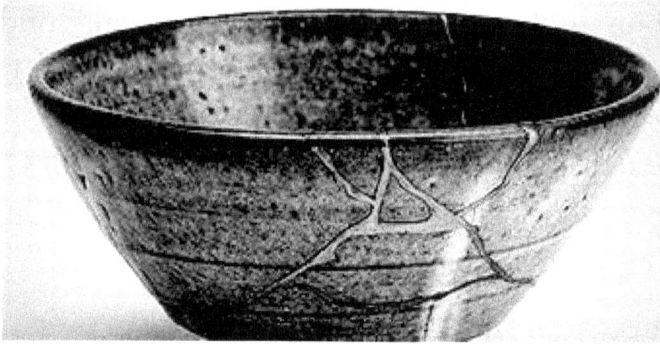

Lastly, Kintsugi is a centuries-old Japanese art of repairing broken pottery. The name of the technique is derived from the words "Kin" (golden) and "tsugi" (joinery), which translates to mean "golden repair."

Kintsugi is the Japanese art of putting broken pottery pieces back together with gold — built on the idea that by embracing flaws and imperfections, you can create an even stronger, more beautiful piece of art. Every break is unique, and instead of repairing an item like new, this technique actually highlights the "scars" as a part of the design. Using this as a metaphor for healing ourselves teaches us an important lesson: Sometimes, in the process of repairing things that have broken, we actually create something more unique, beautiful, and resilient.

It is interesting that Jesus' post-resurrection body bore scars of what He had been through. When Thomas doubted Jesus' resurrection, Jesus invited him to touch the wounds that brought healing to the world. "Put your finger here; see my hands. Reach out your hand and put it into my side" (John 20:27). This is our example. We, also, can offer our wounds to a scarred and scared world for the healing of others—and ultimately ourselves.

CHAPTER TEN

SUMMARY

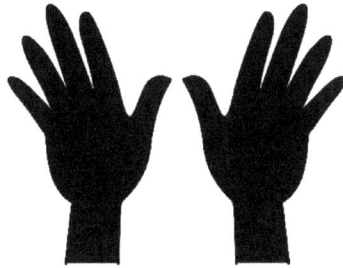

The Bible plainly teaches that adversity can produce beneficial results. Even Jesus, the Son of God, "learned obedience by the things which He suffered. And having been perfected, He became the author of eternal salvation to all who obey Him" (Hebrews 5:8-9).

God reveals that suffering carries with it a noble purpose: It should help us to grow in brotherly love. Paul writes, "Bear one another's burdens, and so fulfill the law of Christ" (Galatians 6:2). When our concern flows out toward others, suffering, as undesirable and painful as it is, can be a catalyst for growth.

The world teaches the idea that suffering or any painful experience is unfair and must be avoided. We live in a quick-fix society that teaches that we do not have to do the hard work to lose weight, get fit, or get through difficult times; we merely have to take a pill for a fast fix to every problem. It is also part of a victim mentality—a refusal to take responsibility for one's behavior or circumstances. This will eventually weaken our society. When we accept that sometimes life is not fair and courageously respond to the challenge -- we grow stronger. The world says that pain is our enemy, an enemy that must be avoided. The world sees no purpose in pain. Trials in our lives can either keep us oppressed or act as an opportunity for growth.

The Bible tells us that God allows suffering to serve divine purposes.

1. Proverbs 16:4 says, "The LORD has made everything for its purpose, even the wicked, for the day of trouble." God has a plan for the world, believers and non-believers. God is a Spirit. Christians are His voice, hands, and feet to complete His purpose here on earth. You can be a part of that plan willingly, or you can disobey His calling. One way or another, God's plan will prevail. Your participation determines how much pain you will be required to endure. When you submit to God's plan, you have the promise that God will be there with you, helping you through your pain. When you are through the trial, I guarantee that you come out of it better than before – God works everything for the good!

2. God sometimes allows us to suffer because pain teaches us to refrain from sin. Discipline is required for our wrong choices. Discipline is actually an act of mercy. Why? Because the consequence of continuing in sin is death (Romans 6:23). Discipline is better than death. Discipline teaches proper behavior. Psalm 119:67 says, "Before I was afflicted, I went astray, but now I keep Your word." King David

reminds us that suffering is a reminder of the consequences of sin and that suffering can produce long-term benefits while we deal with our physical or emotional pain. Emotional and physical pain is often the result of breaking God's commandments, knowingly or unknowingly. We reap what we sow; often, the painful consequences are not immediately felt. "The Lord disciplines those whom he loves, and chastises every child whom he accepts" (Hebrews 12:6).

3. The Bible tells many stories of how God allows adversity to show His love, power, and glory. God has a plan and purpose for everyone, good and bad. The primary plan is to bring *all people* to repentance. Often this requires a painful trial to bring one to repentance. Those He predestines to participate in this plan are often subjected to pain and/or suffering. He may use a bad person or a good person as part of the plan. For example, Daniel in the lion's den, Joseph in slavery, and even Jesus' crucifixion were part of God's plan, who were required to suffer for the greater good. When non-believers see God's work in you, they will also see Jesus in you.

4. Your testimony is a very powerful tool. Your testimony is simply a story – your story of what God has done in your life. Trials in your life give testimonies of God's power and goodness. Without a painful event, there would be no testimony. When you tell others of the wonderful way God brought you through an overwhelming life event, you provide them evidence that we have a loving God, believers

increase their faith, and non-believers have a seed planted. It is God's will to give your testimony of comfort, deliverance, redemption, and salvation. King David shows this in Psalm 105:2, which says, "Sing to Him [God], sing praises to Him; tell of all His wondrous works!"

5. God allows trials in our lives to bring us closer to Him. A painful trial often drives us closer to our creator. Suffering often forces us to examine ourselves and refocuses our priorities and direction to see what is truly important in life. This often forces us to make adjustments and reset priorities, and hopefully, repent bringing us closer to God. We seek comfort in God's love. As we go through the pain of a trial, we learn to lean on God and trust Him to deliver us from the pain, and we draw closer to Him. As we draw closer to God, we recognize the blessings in our lives; we realize God's love.

6. God sometimes allows us to suffer to humble or refine us. Suffering may occur not as a result of sin per se, but because God sees a need to refine and strengthen a part of our character. Peter writes of the value of trials when he explains, "In this, you greatly rejoice, though now for a little while you may have had to suffer grief in all kinds of trials. These have come so that your faith—of greater worth than gold, which perishes even though refined by fire—may be proved genuine and may result in praise, glory, and honor when Jesus Christ is revealed" (1 Peter 1:6-7). These trial-by-fire situations are the catalyst to make the changes God intends.

7. The Bible teaches us that we are merely temporary visitors on this earth. At Jesus' second coming, Christians will be taken to their eternal home – heaven. The reason God does not want us to feel at home on earth is because Satan has control of *the world* (earth). The *world* is a societal system under the control of Satan. We hope for the eternal, non-believers live for the hour. Our goals are different; we seek out doing good. That's why Paul wrote in his letter to the Romans, "Do not be conformed to this world but be transformed by the renewal of your mind, that by testing you may discern what is the will of God, what is good and acceptable and perfect" (v. 12:2). Why not be conformed to the world? Because Paul knows that the world entices *the flesh*. This battle between *the flesh* and *the Spirit* is epic. What is the flesh? Paul doesn't mean our flesh and blood bodies. The flesh is our inner man, which is trained in rebellion by the world and Satan and will battle against us until we experience God's final antidote to the flesh - a resurrection body. The Spirit is the Holy Spirit that is given to all born-again Christians. So, we have a battle against good and evil. This battle causes inner turmoil that oppresses us and keeps us in pain until we repent.

A pain-free life is impossible. We need to face the reality that God can teach us valuable lessons through our suffering. This does not mean suffering will ever be pleasant. Even if we had the opportunity to prepare for the pain in advance, when it actually arrives, we realize that we can never really prepare for the suffering. Pain injects itself into our lives with intense reality. However, suffering prepares us for God's purpose and His

Kingdom. After the trial, we often see God's fingerprints all over it and understand the spiritual maturity it can produce in us. The only escape from the pain comes from God, often when you have achieved the work He intended.

We as humans, consistently blame God for all the evil and suffering in the world. But it is not God who is to blame; the responsibility rests squarely on humans for our decision to reject His guidance and choose a life of disobedience.

The good news is that God knows that our default setting is wanting to do our will. Even after all the disappointment that we cause, He has not given up on mankind. He has given us free will to either follow Him or to go our own way. God allows mankind to suffer to teach us that we cannot find lasting peace, security, and contentment without Him.

Since the fall, God has been allowing people to navigate this life in spiritual darkness. But because we feel that we can rule over our own lives, unless we are in Christ, we cannot succeed. God will bring all people to realize they cannot achieve world peace and bring an end to misery and suffering without His intervention. Our Creator will not allow an evil world to continue indefinitely. He will not allow us to annihilate ourselves. When the time is right, He will send Jesus to earth to rule as King of Kings (Revelation 19:16).

We cannot avoid suffering in a world full of evil, but we should not be discouraged, but have hope knowing that our suffering has a purpose. God is sovereign and ultimately in charge. His promise is to liberate the world from suffering when Christ returns to establish His Kingdom.

No matter the reason for the trial, Jesus promises that He will be by your side every step of the way. One last story, around 605 B.C., King Nebuchadnezzar conquered Jerusalem and took thousands of Jews as slaves. Before the king gave his life to the LORD, he built a large golden idol of himself so that his people could worship him. The golden image was built as a symbol of the king's power and glory.

He commanded his people to bow down and worship the idol. Those who disobeyed would be burned to death in a large furnace. Three of the Jewish slaves refused to bow down to this golden idol that represented a human. Their names were Shadrach, Meshach, and Abednego. They told the King they would only worship God.

The King became angry and ordered the men to be killed in the furnace. The King ordered the furnace to heat up seven times hotter than normal. The guards tied the three men up with rope and threw them in the furnace. The fire was so hot that one of the guards was killed as he was at the door.

King Nebuchadnezzar looked into the fire and said, "Did we not cast three men bound in the fire?" they answered and said to the King, "True, O King." The King responded, "...I see four men unbound walking in the midst of the fire, and they are not hurt; and the appearance of the fourth is like the son of the gods" (Daniel 3:24-25).

The King called the men to come out of the furnace. They came out unbound, unharmed, with no burn smell on their clothing. Needless to say, this made an impression on the King, who declared,

> "Nebuchadnezzar answered and said, 'Blessed be the God of Shadrach, Meshach, and Abednego, who has sent his angel and delivered his servants, who trusted in him, and set aside the king's command, and yielded up their bodies rather than serve and worship any god except their own God. Therefore I make a decree: Any people, nation, or language that speaks anything against the God of Shadrach, Meshach, and Abednego shall be torn limb from limb, and their houses laid in ruins, for there is no other god who is able to rescue in this way.'" --Daniel 3:28-29

Jesus was present in the fire with the three men making sure they came out of their trial-by-fire better than before. This is the promise God makes to his children,

> "But now thus says the LORD, he who created you, O Jacob, he who formed you, O Israel: "Fear not, for I have redeemed you; I have called you by name, you are mine. When you pass through the waters, I will be with you; and through the rivers, they shall not overwhelm you; when you walk through fire, you shall not be burned, and the flame shall not consume you." --Isaiah 43:1-2

There will always be trouble in life, but trust in Jesus, and He will bring you through the difficult times better than before (John 16:33).

I hope and pray that this book has given you some insight into the question of why God allows suffering.

About the Author

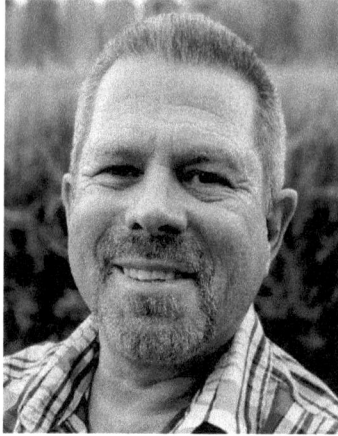

NORM WIELSCH was a law enforcement officer for over twenty-five years. Sixteen of those as an undercover narcotic agent. He experienced many critical incidents during his career. In 1998, he was diagnosed with PTSD and an incurable neuro-muscular disease that caused the loss of feeling, mobility, and strength in his hands and feet. After over thirty surgeries he became addicted to opioids. Due to his sinful responses to his trauma, Norm made a series of poor decisions that landed him in federal prison. It was during the most intense trial of his life that he answered the calling of God who was calling him to minister to people who were suffering from trauma. While in prison, he obtained a master's degree in Theology, a Doctorate Degree in Christian Counseling, and a Drug and Alcohol Counseling Certificate. Norm counseled inmates, preached God's word, taught bible studies. Norm Counseled many inmates who were slaves to their sin. They experienced God's healing power and transformation through the biblical principles taught through Christ-Centered Healing process. Norm is working as an Alcohol and Drug Addiction Counselor and doing pastoral care.

Norm was a police academy instructor and is an expert in PTSD, police tactics, narcotic enforcement, and the first responder culture.

Go to www.Christ-CenteredHealing.com or @ChristCenteredHealing on Facebook to book Norm for your church or other speaking event.

To learn more about Norm and his works scan this QR code: